The Psychiatric Interview

Evaluation and Diagnosis

Expanded from *Psychiatry*, Third Edition, edited by Allan Tasman, Jerald Kay, Jeffrey A. Lieberman, Michael B. First and Mario Maj.

The Psychiatric Interview

Evaluation and Diagnosis

Allan Tasman
Professor and Chair,
Department of Psychiatry and Behavioral Sciences,
University of Louisville School of Medicine,
Louisville, KN,
USA

Jerald Kay
Professor and Chair,
Department of Psychiatry,
Boonshoft School of Medicine, Wright State University,
Dayton, OH,
USA

Robert J. Ursano
Professor and Chair,
Department of Psychiatry,
Uniformed Services University of the Health Sciences,
Bethesda, MD,
USA

WILEY-BLACKWELL
A John Wiley & Sons, Ltd., Publication

This edition first published 2013

Registered Office
John Wiley & Sons, Ltd, The Atrium, Southern Gate, Chichester, West Sussex, PO19 8SQ, UK

Editorial Offices
9600 Garsington Road, Oxford, OX4 2DQ, UK
The Atrium, Southern Gate, Chichester, West Sussex, PO19 8SQ, UK
111 River Street, Hoboken, NJ 07030-5774, USA

For details of our global editorial offices, for customer services and for information about how to apply for permission to reuse the copyright material in this book please see our website at www.wiley.com/wiley-blackwell.

Library of Congress Cataloging-in-Publication Data

The psychiatric interview : evaluation and diagnosis / [edited by] Allan Tasman, Jerald Kay, Robert J. Ursano.
p. ; cm.
Includes bibliographical references and index.
ISBN 978-1-118-34097-4 (epdf) – ISBN 978-1-118-34098-1 (epub) – ISBN 978-1-118-34099-8 (emobi) – ISBN 978-1-118-34100-1 (obook) – ISBN 978-1-119-97623-3 (cloth : alk. paper)
I. Tasman, Allan, 1947– II. Kay, Jerald. III. Ursano, Robert J., 1947–
[DNLM: 1. Interview, Psychological–methods. 2. Ethics, Professional. 3. Mental Disorders–diagnosis. 4. Physician-Patient Relations. WM 143]
616.89′075–dc23

2012050615

A catalogue record for this book is available from the British Library.

Wiley also publishes its books in a variety of electronic formats. Some content that appears in print may not be available in electronic books.

Cover image: © iStockphoto/Henry Chaplin
Cover design by Grounded Design

Set in 10/12pt Times by SPi Publisher Services, Pondicherry, India
Printed and bound in Malaysia by Vivar Printing Sdn Bhd

1 2013

Contents

Contributors

Deborah L. Cabaniss
Department of Psychiatry,
Columbia University College of
Physicians and Surgeons,
New York, NY,
USA
New York State Psychiatric Institute,
New York, NY,
USA

Kenneth Certa
Department of Psychiatry
and Human Behavior,
Thomas Jefferson University,
Philadelphia, PA,
USA

Francine Cournos
New York State Psychiatric Institute,
New York, NY,
USA

Allison Cowan
Department of Psychiatry,
Boonshoft School of Medicine,
Wright State University,
Dayton, OH,
USA

Richard S. Epstein
F. Edward Hébert School of Medicine,
Uniformed Services University
of the Health Sciences,
Bethesda, MD,
USA

Jaswant Guzder
Division of Social and Transcultural
Psychiatry,
McGill University,
Montreal, Quebec,
Canada

G. Eric Jarvis
Division of Social and Transcultural
Psychiatry,
McGill University,
Montreal, Quebec,
Canada

Abigail Kay
Department of Psychiatry and Human
Behavior,
Thomas Jefferson University,
Philadelphia, PA,
USA

Jerald Kay
Department of Psychiatry,
Boonshoft School of Medicine,
Wright State University,
Dayton, OH,
USA

Laurence J. Kirmayer
Division of Social and Transcultural
Psychiatry,
McGill University,
Montreal, Quebec,
Canada

David A. Lowenthal
New York State Psychiatric Institute,
New York, NY,
USA

Paul C. Mohl
Department of Psychiatry,
University of Texas Southwestern
Medical Center,
Dallas, TX,
USA

Ahmed Okasha
WHO Collaborating Center for Research
and Training in Mental Health,
Ain Shams University,
Cairo,
Egypt

Cécile Rousseau
Division of Social and Transcultural
Psychiatry,
McGill University,
Montreal, Quebec,
Canada

Edward K. Silberman
Department of Psychiatry,
Tufts University,
Boston, MA,
USA

Stephen M. Sonnenberg
Department of Psychiatry,
Uniformed Services University
of the Health Sciences,
Bethesda, MD,
USA

Amy M. Ursano
Department of Psychiatry,
University of North Carolina,
Chapel Hill, NC,
USA

Robert J. Ursano
Department of Psychiatry,
Uniformed Services University
of the Health Sciences,
Bethesda, MD,
USA

Randon Welton
Department of Psychiatry,
Boonshoft School of Medicine,
Wright State University,
Dayton, OH,
USA
PTSD Program,
Dayton Veterans Administrative Hospital,
Dayton, OH,
USA

Preface

The tools of diagnosis in psychiatry, as is true for all of medicine, have vastly improved in the past decades. We now can image the brain to look at structures, see changes in the brain with development, identify functional areas of the brain as they are operating, and measure blood levels of hormones and medications. All of these allow us to better assess and care for our patients. Although these have been remarkable advances, the patient interview and the evolving doctor–patient relationship continue to provide the setting and the structure to gather core data to begin assessment and treatment in all of medicine and especially in psychiatry. This is true regardless of the clinical setting, whether inpatient, outpatient, consultation/liaison, the emergency department, or telepsychiatry. This book provides both the information needed to conduct an in-depth psychiatric evaluation as well as a thorough discussion of how to begin forming and maintaining the therapeutic alliance. The heart of the philosophy embodied in this work is that we must learn who is the person with the illness, as well as what is the illness, and why it appeared, reappeared, or continues, in order to maintain the treatment relationship most likely to produce a positive clinical outcome. The strengthening of this relationship and assuring the best treatment is facilitated through the development of a case formulation which also is addressed in depth within the book.

The clinical interview is the process of listening to and understanding the patient, and effectively communicating that understanding within the context of the doctor–patient relationship. How to conduct an interview to maximize discerning the most important information while developing and maintaining the best long-term relationship on which to build treatment is the goal of this book. Interviewing requires knowing how to listen for information often outside of the patient's awareness, how to communicate, how to maintain the therapeutic relationship, and appreciate the dynamic, interpersonal, cultural, and ethical issues central to the clinical process. The advances in both understanding the effect of development on the patient's capacities to form meaningful relationships and the improved diagnostic systems used to recognize specific psychopathology have helped improve the clinician's assessment of the varying degrees of the individual patient's pre-existing capability to trust the physician. The ability to discern these limitations alerts the interviewer to the need to tailor the style of the interview for each patient in order to maximize the success of a multimodal treatment plan.

We believe this book will be of particular importance for students, postgraduate trainees, and those in the early stages of their careers. But we also know that no matter what the stage of a clinician's career, the material in this book will serve as a useful guide and reference. We hope you find this book as useful to your practice as we have found it gratifying to prepare.

Allan Tasman
Jerald Kay
Robert J. Ursano

Acknowledgments

The editors would like to extend their gratitude to the contributors of the third edition of *Psychiatry*, on which some of this book is based. They would also like to thank Paul C. Mohl, Laurence J. Kirmayer, Cécile Rousseau, G. Eric Jarvis, Jaswant Guzder, Edward K. Silberman, Kenneth Certa, Abigail Kay, Richard S. Epstein, Ahmed Okasha, Amy M. Ursano, Stephen M. Sonnenberg, Robert J. Ursano, Francine Cournos, David A. Lowenthal, and Deborah L. Cabaniss.

CHAPTER

1 Listening to the Patient

Listening: The Key Skill in Psychiatry

It was Freud who raised the psychiatric technique of examination – listening – to a level of expertise unexplored in earlier eras. As Binswanger (1963) has said of the period prior to Freudian influence: psychiatric "auscultation" and "percussion" of the patient was performed as if through the patient's shirt with so much of his essence remaining covered or muffled that layers of meaning remained unpeeled away or unexamined.

This metaphor and parallel to the cardiac examination is one worth considering as we first ask if listening will remain as central a part of psychiatric examination as in the past. The explosion of biomedical knowledge has radically altered our evolving view and practice of the doctor–patient relationship. Physicians of an earlier generation were taught that the diagnosis is made at the bedside – that is, the history and physical examination are paramount. Laboratory and imaging (radiological, in those days) examinations were seen as confirmatory exercises. However, as our technologies have blossomed, the bedside and/or consultation room examinations have evolved into the method whereby the physician determines what tests to run, and the tests are often viewed as making the diagnosis. So can one imagine a time in the not-too-distant future when the psychiatrist's task will be to identify that the patient is psychotic and then order some benign brain imaging study which will identify the patient's exact disorder?

Perhaps so, but will that obviate the need for the psychiatrist's special kind of listening? Indeed, there are those who claim that psychiatrists should no longer be considered experts in the doctor–patient relationship, where expertise is derived from their unique training in listening skills, but experts in the brain. As we come truly to understand the relationship between brain states and subtle cognitive, emotional, and interpersonal states, one could also ask if this is a distinction that really makes a difference. On the other hand, the psychiatrist will always be charged with finding a way to relate effectively to those who cannot effectively relate to themselves or to others. There is something in the treatment of individuals whose illnesses express themselves through disturbances of thinking, feeling, perceiving, and behaving that will always demand special expertise in establishing a therapeutic relationship – and that is dependent on special expertise in listening (Clinical Vignette 1).

All psychiatrists, regardless of theoretical stance, must learn this skill and struggle with how it is to be defined and taught. The biological or phenomenological psychiatrist

---

The Psychiatric Interview: Evaluation and Diagnosis, First Edition. Allan Tasman, Jerald Kay and Robert J. Ursano.

This chapter is based on Chapter 1 (Paul C. Mohl) of *Psychiatry*, 3rd Edition.

Clinical Vignette 1

A 28-year-old white married man suffering from paranoid schizophrenia and obsessive–compulsive disorder did extremely well in the hospital, where his medication had been changed to clozapine with good effects. But he rapidly deteriorated on his return home. It was clear that the ward milieu had been a crucial part of his improvement, so partial hospitalization was recommended. The patient demurred, saying he didn't want to be a "burden". The psychiatrist explored this with the patient and his wife. Beyond the obvious "burdens" of cost and travel arrangements, the psychiatrist detected the patient's striving to be autonomously responsible for handling his illness. By conveying a deep respect for that wish, and then educating the already insightful patient about the realities of "bearing schizophrenia", the psychiatrist was able to help the patient accept the needed level of care.

listens for subtle expressions of symptomatology; the cognitive–behavioral psychiatrist listens for hidden distortions, irrational assumptions, or global inferences; the psychodynamic psychiatrist listens for hints at unconscious conflicts; the behaviorist listens for covert patterns of anxiety and stimulus associations; the family systems psychiatrist listens for hidden family myths and structures.

This requires sensitivity to the storyteller, which integrates a patient orientation complementing a disease orientation. The listener's intent is to uncover what is wrong and to put a label on it. At the same time, the listener is on a journey to discover who the patient is, employing tools of asking, looking, testing, and clarifying. The patient is invited to collaborate as an active informer. Listening work takes time, concentration, imagination, a sense of humor, and an attitude that places the patient as the hero of his or her own life story. Key listening skills are listed in Table 1.1.

Table 1.1 Key Listening Skills

Hearing	Connotative meanings of words
	Idiosyncratic uses of language
	Figures of speech that tell a deeper story
	Voice tones and modulation (e.g., hard edge, voice cracking)
	Stream of associations
Seeing	Posture
	Gestures
	Facial expressions (e.g., eyes watering, jaw clenched)
	Other outward expressions of emotion
Comparing	Noting what is omitted
	Dissonances between modes of expression
	Intuiting
Reflecting	Attending to one's own internal reactions
	Thinking it all through outside the immediate pressure to respond during the interview

The enduring art of psychiatry involves guiding the depressed patient, for example, to tell his or her story of loss in addition to having him or her name, describe, and quantify symptoms of depression. The listener, in hearing the story, experiences the world and the patient from the patient's point of view and helps carry the burden of loss, lightening and transforming the load. In hearing the sufferer, the depression itself is lifted and relieved. The listening is healing as well as diagnostic. If done well, the listener becomes a better disease diagnostician. The best listeners hear both the patient and the disease clearly, and regard every encounter as potentially therapeutic.

The Primary Tools: Words, Analogies, Metaphors, Similes, and Symbols

To listen and understand requires that the language used between the speaker and the hearer be shared – that the meanings of words and phrases are commonly held. Patients are storytellers who have the hope of being heard and understood. Their hearers are physicians who expect to listen actively and to be with the patient in a new level of understanding. Because all human beings listen to so many different people every day, we tend to think of listening as an automatic ongoing process, yet this sort of active listening remains one of the central skills in clinical psychiatry. It underpins all other skills in diagnosis, alliance building, and communication. In all medical examinations, the patient is telling a story only she or he has experienced. The physician must glean the salient information and then use it in appropriate ways. Inevitably, even when language is common, there are subtle differences in meanings, based upon differences in gender, age, culture, religion, socioeconomic class, race, region of upbringing, nationality and original language, as well as the idiosyncrasies of individual history. These differences are particularly important to keep in mind in the use of analogies, similes, and metaphors. Figures of speech, in which one thing is held representational of another by comparison, are very important windows to the inner world of the patient. Differences in meanings attached to these figures of speech can complicate their use. In psychodynamic assessment and psychotherapeutic treatment, the need to regard these subtleties of language becomes the self-conscious focus of the psychiatrist, yet failure to hear and heed such idiosyncratic distinctions can affect simple medical diagnosis as well (Clinical Vignettes 2 and 3).

Clinical Vignette 2

A psychiatric consultant was asked to see a 48-year-old man on a coronary care unit for chest pain deemed "functional" by the cardiologist who had asked the patient if his chest pain was "crushing". The patient said no. A variety of other routine tests were also negative. The psychiatrist asked the patient to describe his pain. He said, "It's like a truck sitting on my chest, squeezing it down". The psychiatrist promptly recommended additional tests, which confirmed the diagnosis of myocardial infarction. The cardiologist may have been tempted to label the patient a "bad historian", but the most likely culprit of this potentially fatal misunderstanding lies in the connotative meanings, each ascribed to the word "crushing" or to other variances in metaphorical communication.

Clinical Vignette 3

A psychiatrist had been treating a 35-year-old man with a narcissistic personality and dysthymic disorder for 2 years. Given the brutality and deprivation of the patient's childhood, the clinician was persistently puzzled by the patient's remarkable psychological strengths. He possessed capacities for empathy, self-observation, and modulation of intense rage that were unusual, given his background. During a session, the patient, in telling a childhood story, began, "When I was a little fella…". It struck the psychiatrist that the patient always said "little fella" when referring to himself as a boy, and that this was fairly distinctive phraseology. Almost all other patients will say, "When I was young/a kid/a girl (boy)/in school", designate an age, etc. On inquiry about this, the patient immediately identified "The Andy Griffith Show" as the source. This revealed a secret identification with the characters of the TV show, and a model that said to a young boy, "There are other ways to be a man than what you see around you". Making this long-standing covert identification fully conscious was transformative for the patient.

In psychotherapy, the special meanings of words become the central focus of the treatment.

How Does One Hear Words in This Way?

The preceding clinical vignettes, once described, sound straightforward and easy. Yet, to listen in this way, the clinician must acquire specific yet difficult-to-learn skills and attitudes. It is extremely difficult to put into words the listening processes embodied in these examples and those to follow, yet that is what this chapter attempts to do.

Students, when observing experienced psychiatrists interviewing patients, often express a sense of wonder such as: "How did she know to ask that?" "Why did the patient open up with him but not with me?" "What made the diagnosis so clear in that interview and not in all the others?" The student may respond with a sense of awe, a feeling of ineptitude and doubt at ever achieving such facility, or even a reaction of disparagement that the process seems so indefinable and inexact. The key is the clinician's ability to listen. Without a refined capacity to hear deeply, the chapters on other aspects of interviewing in this textbook are of little use. But it is neither mystical nor magical nor indefinable (though it is very difficult to articulate); such skills are the product of hard work, much thought, intense supervision, and extensive in-depth exposure to many different kinds of patients.

Psychiatrists, more than any other physicians, must simultaneously listen symptomatically and narratively/experientially. They must also have access to a variety of theoretical perspectives that effectively inform their listening. These include behavioral, interpersonal, cognitive, sociocultural, and systems theories. Symptomatic listening is what we think of as traditional medical history taking, in which the focus is on the presence or absence of a particular symptom, the most overt content level of an interview. Narrative–experiential listening is based on the idea that all humans are constantly interpreting their experiences, attributing meaning to them, and weaving a story of their lives with themselves as the central character. This process goes on continuously, both consciously and unconsciously, as a running conversation within each of us. The conversation is between parts of ourselves and between ourselves and what Freud called "internalized objects", important people in our lives whose images, sayings, and attitudes become permanently laid down in our memories. This conversation and commentary on our lives includes personal history, repetitive behaviors, learned assumptions about the world, and interpersonal roles. These are, in turn, the products of individual background, cultural norms and values, national identifications, spiritual meanings, and family system forces (Clinical Vignette 4).

Clinical Vignette 4

A 46-year-old man was referred to a psychiatrist from a drug study. The patient had both major depression and dysthymic disorder since a business failure 2 years earlier. His primary symptoms were increased sleep and decreased mood, libido, energy, and interests. After no improvement during the "blind" portion of the study, he had continued to show little response once the code was broken, and he was treated with two different active antidepressant medications. He was referred for psychotherapy and further antidepressant trials. The therapy progressed slowly with only episodic improvement. One day, the patient reported that his wife had been teasing him about how, during his afternoon nap, his snoring could be heard over the noise of a vacuum cleaner. The psychiatrist immediately asked additional questions, eventually obtained sleep polysomnography, and, after appropriate treatment for sleep apnea, the patient's depression improved dramatically.

It seems that three factors were present that enabled the psychiatrist in Clinical Vignette 4 to listen well and identify an unusual diagnosis that had been missed by at least three other excellent clinicians who had all been using detailed structured interviews that were extremely inclusive in their symptom reviews. First, the psychiatrist had to have readily available in mind all sorts of symptoms and syndromes. Second, he had to be in a curious mode. In fact, this clinician had a gnawing sense that something was missing in his understanding of the patient. There is a saying in American medicine designed to focus students on the need to consider common illnesses first, while not totally ignoring rarer diseases: when you hear hoofbeats in the road, don't look first for zebras. We would say that this psychiatrist's mind was open to seeing a "zebra" despite the ongoing assumption that the weekly "hoofbeats" he had been hearing represented the everyday "horse" of clinical depression. Finally, he had to hear the patient's story in multiple, flexible ways, including the possibility that a symptom may be embedded in it, so that a match could be noticed between a detail of the story and a symptom. Eureka! The zebra could then be seen although it had been standing there every week for months.

Looking back at Clinical Vignette 3, we see the same phenomenon of a detail leaping out as a significant piece of missing information that dramatically influences the treatment process. To accomplish this requires a cognitive template (symptoms and syndromes; developmental, systemic, and personality theories; awareness of cultural perspectives), a searching curious stance, and flexible processing of the data presented. If one is able to internalize the skills listed in Table 1.1, the listener begins automatically to hear the meanings in the words.

Listening as More Than Hearing

Listening and hearing are often equated in many people's minds. However, listening involves not only hearing and understanding the speaker's words, but attending to inflection, metaphor, imagery, sequence of associations, and interesting linguistic selections. It also involves seeing – movement, gestures, facial expressions, subtle changes in these – and constantly comparing what is said with what is seen, looking for dissonances, and comparing what is being said and seen with what was previously communicated and observed. Further, it is essential to be aware of what might have been said but was not, or how things might have been expressed but were not. This is where clues to idiosyncratic meanings and associations are often discovered. Sometimes, the most important meanings are embedded in what is conspicuous by its absence.

There appears to be a biogrammar of primary emotions that all humans share and express in predictable, fixed action patterns. The meaning of a smile or nod of the head is universal across disparate cultures. The amygdala and the inferior temporal lobe gyrus have been identified as the neurobiological substrate for recognition of and empathy for others and their emotional states. Further research has identified that these parts of the brain are, on the one hand, prededicated to recognizing certain gestures, facial expressions, and so on, but require effective maternal–infant interaction in order to do so (Schore, 2001). All of this is synthesized in the listener as a "sense" or intuition as to what the speaker is saying at multiple levels. The availability of useful cognitive templates and theories enables the listener to articulate what is heard (Clinical Vignette 5).

Clinical Vignette 5

A 38-year-old Hispanic construction worker presented himself to a small-town emergency department in the Southwest, complaining of pain on walking, actually described in Spanish-accented English as "a little pain". His voice was tight, his face was drawn, and his physical demeanor was burdened and hesitant. His response to the invitation to walk was met by a labored attempt to walk without favor to his painful limb. A physician could have discharged him from the emergency department with a small prescription of ibuprofen. The careful physician in the emergency department responded to the powerful visual message that he was in pain, was beaten down by it, and had suffered long before coming in. This recognition came first to the physician as an intuition that this man was somehow more sick than he made himself sound. A radiograph of the femur revealed a lytic lesion that later proved to be metastatic renal cell carcinoma. To hear the unspoken, one had to be keenly aware of the patient's tone and how he looked, and to keep in mind, too, the cultural taboos forbidding him to give in to pain or to appear to need help.

As has been implied, not only must one affirmatively "hear" all that a patient is communicating, one must overcome a variety of potential blocks to effective listening.

Common Blocks to Effective Listening

Many factors influence the ability to listen. Psychiatrists come to the patient as the product of their own life experiences. Does the listener tune in to what he or she hears in a more attentive way if the listener and the patient share characteristics? What blocks to listening (Table 1.2) are posed by differences in sex, age, religion, socioeconomic class, race, culture, or nationality? What blind spots may be induced by superficial similarities in different personal meanings attributed to the same cultural symbol? Separate and apart from the differences in the development of empathy when the dyad holds in common certain features, the act of listening is inevitably influenced by similarities and differences between the psychiatrist and the patient.

Table 1.2 Blocks to Effective Listening

Patient–psychiatrist dissimilarities	Race Sex Culture Religion Regional dialect Individual differences Socioeconomic class
Superficial similarities	May lead to incorrect assumptions of shared meanings
Countertransference	Psychiatrist fails to hear or reacts inappropriately to content reminiscent of own unresolved conflicts
External forces	Managed care setting Emergency department Control-oriented inpatient unit
Attitudes	Need for control Psychiatrist having a bad day

Would a woman have reported the snoring in Clinical Vignette 4 or would she have been too embarrassed? Would she have reported it more readily to a woman psychiatrist? What about the image in Clinical Vignette 2 of a truck sitting on someone's chest? How gender and culture bound is it? Would "The Andy Griffith Show", important in Clinical Vignette 3, have had the same impact on a young African-American boy that it did on a Caucasian one? In how many countries is "The Andy Griffith Show" even available, and in which cultures would that model of a family structure seem relevant? Suppose the psychiatrist in that vignette was not a television viewer or had come from another country to the USA long after the show had come and gone? Consider these additional examples (Clinical Vignette 6).

Clinical Vignette 6

A female patient came to see her male psychiatrist for their biweekly session. Having just been given new duties on her job, she came in excitedly and began sharing with her therapist how happy she was to have been chosen by her male supervisor to help him with a very important project at their office. The session continued with the theme of the patient's pride in having been recognized for her attributes, talents, and hard work. At the next session, she said that she had become embarrassed after the previous session at the thought that she had been "strutting her stuff". The therapist reflected back to her the thought that she sounded like a rooster strutting his stuff, connecting her embarrassment at having revealed that she strove for the recognition and power of men in her company, and that she, in fact, envied the position of her supervisor. The patient objected to the comparison of a rooster, and likened it more to feeling like a woman of the streets strutting her stuff. She stated that she felt like a prostitute being used by her supervisor. The psychiatrist was off the mark by missing the opportunity to point out in the analogous way that the patient's source of embarrassment was in being used, not so much in being envious of the male position.

It is likely that different life experiences based on gender fostered this misunderstanding. How many women easily identify with the stereotyped role of the barnyard rooster? How many men readily identify with the role of a prostitute? These are but two examples of the myriad different meanings our specific gender may incline us toward. Although metaphor is a powerful tool in listening to the patient, cross-cultural barriers pose potential blocks to understanding (Clinical Vignettes 7 and 8).

Clinical Vignette 7

A 36-year-old black woman complained to her therapist (of the same language, race, and socioeconomic class) that her husband was a snake, meaning that he was no good, treacherous, a hidden danger. The therapist, understanding this commonly held definition of a snake, reflected back to the patient pertinent, supportive feedback concerning the care and caution the patient was exercising in divorce dealings with the husband.

In contrast, a 36-year-old Chinese woman, fluent in English, living in her adopted country for 15 years and assimilated to Western culture, represented her husband to her Caucasian, native-born psychiatrist as being like a dragon. The therapist, without checking on the meaning of the word "dragon" with her patient, assumed it connoted danger, one of malicious intent and oppression. The patient, however, was using "dragon" as a metaphor for her husband – the fierce, watchful guardian of the family – in keeping with the ancient Chinese folklore in which the dragon is stationed at the gates of the lord's castle to guard and protect it from evil and danger.

Clinical Vignette 8

In a family session, a psychiatrist from the South referred to the mother of her patient as "your mama", intending a meaning of warmth and respect. The patient instantly became enraged at the use of such an offensive term toward her mother. Although being treated in Texas, the patient and her family had recently moved from a large city in New Jersey. The use of the term "mama" among working-class Italians in that area was looked upon with derision among people of Irish descent, the group to which the patient was ethnically connected. The patient had used the term "mother" to refer to her mother, a term the psychiatrist had heard with a degree of coolness attached. What she knew of her patient's relationship with her mother did not fit in with a word like mother; hence, almost out of awareness, she switched terms, leading to a response of indignation and outrage from the patient.

Even more subtle regional variations may produce similar problems in listening and understanding.

Psychiatrists discern meaning in that which they hear through filters of their own – cultural backgrounds, life experiences, feelings, the day's events, their own physical sense of themselves, nationality, sex roles, religious meaning systems, and intrapsychic conflicts. The filters can serve as blocks or as magnifiers if certain elements of what is being said resonate with something within the psychiatrist. When the filters block, we call it countertransference or insensitivity. When they magnify, we call it empathy or sensitivity. One may observe a theme for a long time repeated with a different tone, embellishment, inflection, or context before the idea of what is meant comes to mind. The "little fella" example in Clinical Vignette 3 illustrates a message that had been communicated in many ways and times in exactly the same language before the psychiatrist "got it". On discovering a significant meaning that had been signaled previously in many ways, the psychiatrist often has the experience: "How could I have been so stupid? It's been staring me in the face for months!"

Managed care and the manner in which national health systems are administered can alter our attitudes toward the patient and our abilities to be transforming listeners. The requirement for authorization for minimal visits, time on the phone with utilization review nurses attempting to justify continuing therapy, and forms tediously filled out can be blocks to listening to the patient. Limitations on the kinds and length of treatment can lull the psychiatrist into not listening in the same way or as intently. With these time limits and other "third-party payer" considerations (i.e., need for a billable diagnostic code), the psychiatrist, as careful listener, must heed the external pressures influencing the approach to the patient. Many health benefit packages will provide coverage in any therapeutic setting only for relief of symptoms, restoration of minimal function, acute problem solving, and shoring up of defenses. In various countries, health-care systems have come up with a variety of constraints in their efforts to deal with the costs of care. Unless these pressures are attended to, listening will be accomplished with a different purpose in mind, more closely approximating the crisis intervention model of the emergency room or the medical model for either inpatient or outpatient care. In these settings, the thoughtful psychiatrist will arm himself or herself with checklists, inventories, and scales for objectifying the severity of illness and response to treatment: the ear is tuned only to measurable and observable signs of responses to therapy and biologic intervention (Clinical Vignette 9).

Clinical Vignette 9

An army private was brought to the emergency room in Germany by his friends, having threatened to commit suicide while holding a gun to his head. He was desperate, disorganized, impulsive, enraged, pacing, and talking almost incoherently. Gradually, primarily through his friends, the story emerged that his first sergeant had recently made a decision for the entire unit that had a particularly adverse effect on the patient. He was a fairly primitive character who relied on his wife for a sense of stability and coherence in his life. The sergeant's decision was to send the entire unit into the field for over a month just at the time the patient's wife was about to arrive, after a long delay, from the USA. After piecing together this story, the psychiatrist said to the patient, "It's not yourself you want to kill, it's your first sergeant!" The patient at first giggled a little, then gradually broke out into a belly laugh that echoed throughout the emergency room. It was clear that, having recognized the true object of his anger, a coherence was restored that enabled him to feel his rage without the impulse to act on it. The psychiatrist then enlisted the friends in a plan to support the patient through the month and to arrange regular phone contact with the wife as she set up their new home in Germany. No medication was necessary. Hospitalization was averted, and a request for humanitarian dispensation, which would have compromised the patient in the eyes of both his peers and superiors, was avoided as well. And, with luck, the young man had an opportunity to grow emotionally as well.

With emphasis on learning here and now symptoms that can bombard the dyad with foreground static and noise, will the patient be lost in the encounter? The same approach to listening occurs in the setting of the emergency department for crisis intervention. Emphasis is on symptom relief, assurance of capacities to keep oneself safe, restoration of minimal function, acute problem solving, and shoring up of defenses. Special attention is paid to identifying particular stressors. What can be done quickly to change stressors that throw the patient's world into a state of disequilibrium? The difference in the emergency room is that the careful listener may have 3–6 hours, as opposed to three to six sessions for the patient with a health maintenance organization or preferred provider contract, or other limitations on benefits. If one is fortunate and good at being an active listener–bargainer, the seeds of change can be planted in the hope of allowing them time to grow between visits to the emergency department. If one could hope for another change, it would be for a decrease in the chaos in the patient's inner world and outer world.

Crucial Attitudes That Enable Effective Listening

The first step in developing good listening skills involves coming to grips with the importance of inner experience in psychiatric treatment and diagnosis. The advent of modern diagnostic classifications has been responsible for enormous advances in reliability and accuracy of diagnosis, but their emphasis on seemingly observable phenomena has allowed the willing user to forget the importance of inner experience even in such basic diagnoses as major depressive disorder. Consider the symptom "depressed mood most of the day" or "markedly diminished interest or pleasure" or even "decrease or increase in appetite". These are entirely subjective symptoms. Simply reporting depression is usually not sufficient to convince a psychiatrist that a diagnosis of depression is warranted. In fact, the vast majority of psychiatric patients are so demoralized by their illnesses that they often announce depression as their first complaint. Further, there are a significant number of patients who do not acknowledge depression yet are so diagnosed. The clinician might well comment: "Sitting with him makes me feel very sad".

The psychiatrist must listen to much more than the patient's overt behavior. There are qualities in the communication, including the inner experiences induced in the listener, that should be attended to. The experienced clinician listens to the words, watches the behavior, engages in and notices the ongoing interaction, allows himself or herself to experience his or her own inner reactions to the process, and *never forgets that depression and almost all other psychiatric symptoms are exclusively private experiences.* The behavior and interactions are useful insofar as they assist the psychiatrist in inferring the patient's inner experience.

Therefore, to convince a clinician that a patient is depressed, not only must the patient say she or he is depressed, but the observable behavior must convey it (sad-looking face, sighing, unexpressive intonations, etc.); the interaction with the interviewer must convey depressive qualities (sense of neediness, sadness induced in the interviewer, beseeching qualities expressed, etc.). In the absence of both of these, other diagnoses should be considered, but in the presence of such qualities, depression needs to remain in the differential diagnosis.

Even when we make statements about brain function with regard to a particular patient, we use this kind of listening, generally, by making at least two inferences. We first listen to and observe the patient and then infer some aspect of the patient's private experience. Then, if we possess sufficient scientific knowledge, we make a second inference to a disturbance in neurochemistry, neurophysiology, or neuroanatomy. When psychiatrists prescribe antidepressant medication, they have inferred from words, moved into inner experiences, and come to a conclusion that there is likely a dysregulation of serotonin or norepinephrine in the patient's brain.

As one moves toward treatment from diagnosis, the content of inner experience inferred may change to more varied states of feelings, needs, and conflicts, but the fundamental process of listening remains the same. The psychiatrist listens for the meaning of all behavior, to the ongoing interpersonal relationship the patient attempts to establish, and to inner experiences as well.

Despite all of the technological advances in medicine in general and their growing presence in psychiatry, securing or eliciting a history remains the first and central skill for all physicians. Even in the most basic of medical situations, the patient is trying to communicate a set of private experiences (how does one describe the qualities of pain or discomfort?) that the physician may infer and sort into possible syndromes and diagnoses. In psychiatry, this process is multiplied, as indicated in Figure 1.1.

It was widely assumed that development, and problems related to development, effect the inner experiences of various affects. Does, for example, a person with borderline personality disorder experience "anxiety" in the same qualitative and quantitative manner in which a neurotic person does? What is the relationship between sadness and

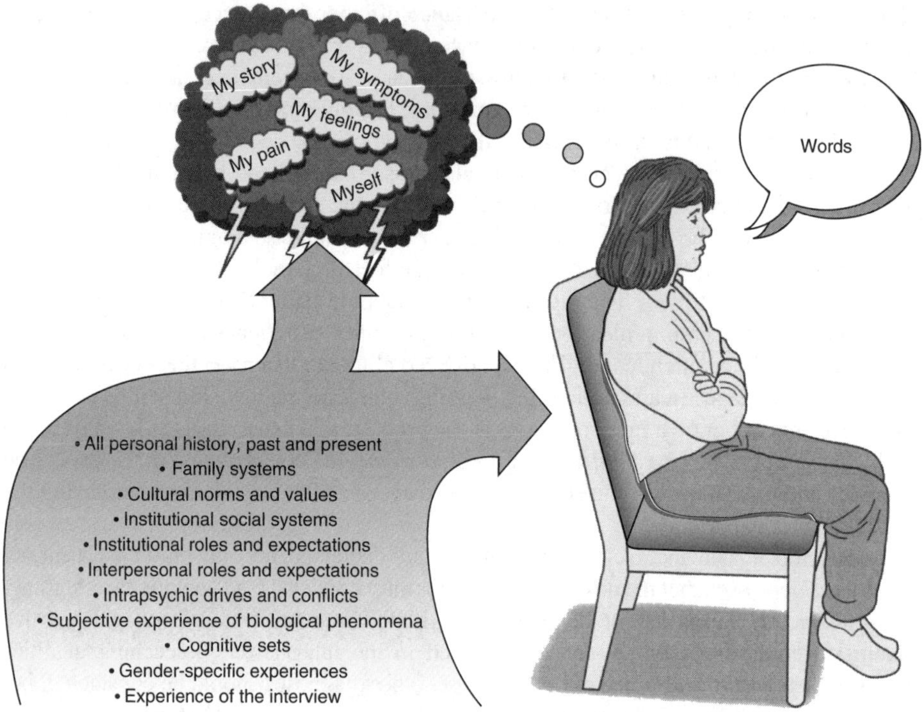

Figure 1.1 *Finding the patient (Kay and Tasman, 2006).*

guilt and the empty experiences of depression? This perspective underlies the principle articulated in text after text on interviewing that emphasizes the importance of establishing rapport in the process of history taking. It is incredibly easy for the psychiatrist to attribute to the patient what she or he would have meant and what most people might have meant in using a particular word or phrase. The sense in the narrator that the listener is truly present, connected, and with the patient enormously enhances the accuracy of the story reported.

Words that have been used to describe this process of constant attention to and inference of inner experience by the listener include interest, empathy, attentiveness, and noncontingent positive regard. However, these are words that may say less than they seem to. It is the constant curious awareness on the listener's part, that she or he is trying to grasp the private inner experience of the patient, and the storyteller's sense of this stance by the psychiatrist that impel the ever more revealing process of history taking. This quality of listening produces what we call rapport, without which psychiatric histories become spotty, superficial, and even suspect. There are no bad historians, only patients who have not yet found the right listener.

It is well established that two powerful predictors of outcome in any form of psychotherapy are empathy and the therapeutic alliance. This has been shown again and again in study after study for dynamic therapy, cognitive therapy, behavior therapy, and even medication management. The truth of this can be seen in the remarkable therapeutic success of the

Table 1.3 Attitudes Important to Listening

The centrality of *inner experience*
There are no bad historians
The answer is always inside the patient
Control and power are shared in the interview
It is OK to feel confused and uncertain
Objective truth is never as simple as it seems
Listen to yourself, too
Everything you hear is modified by the patient's filters
Everything you hear is modified by your own filters
There will always be another opportunity to hear more clearly

"clinical management" cell of the National Institutes of Mental Health Collaborative Study on the Treatment of Major Depression. Although the Clinical Management Cell was not as effective as the cells that included specific drugs or specific psychotherapeutic interventions, 35% of patients with moderate to severe major depressive disorder improved significantly with carefully structured supportive clinical management alone (Elkin *et al.*, 1989).

Helpful psychiatric listening requires a complicated attitude toward control and power in the interview (see Table 1.3). The psychiatrist invites the patient/storyteller to collaborate as an active informer. He or she is invited, too, to question and observe himself or herself. This method of history taking remains the principal tool of general clinical medicine. However, as Freud pointed out, these methods of active uncovering are more complex in the psychic realm. The use of the patient as a voluntary reporter requires that the investigator keep in mind the unconscious and its power over the patient and listener. Can the patient be a reliable objective witness of himself or herself or his or her symptoms? Can the listener hold in mind his or her own set of filters, meanings, and distortions as he or she hears? The listener translates for himself or herself and his or her patient the patient's articulation of his or her experience of himself or herself and his or her inner world into our definition of symptoms, syndromes, and differential diagnoses, which make up the concept of the medical model.

Objective–descriptive examiners are like detectives closing in on disease. The psychiatric detective enters the inquiry with an attitude of unknowing and suspends prior opinion. The techniques of listening invoke a wondering and a wandering with the patient. Periods of head scratching and exclamations of "I'm confused", or "I don't understand", or "That's awful!", or "Tell me more", allow the listener to follow or to point the way for the dyad. Finally, clear and precise descriptions are held up for scrutiny, with the hope that a diagnostic label or new information about the patient's suffering and emotional pain be revealed.

It is embarking on the history taking journey together – free of judgments, opinions, criticism, or preconceived notions – that underpins rapport. Good listening requires a complex understanding of what objective truth is and how it may be found. The effective psychiatrist must eschew the traditional medical role in interviewing and tolerate a collaborative, at times meandering, direction in which control is at best shared and sometimes wholly with the patient. The psychiatrist constantly asks: What is being said? Why is it being said at this moment? What is the meaning of what is being said? In what context is all this emerging? What does that tell me about the meaning of and what does it reflect about the doctor–patient relationship?

Theoretical Perspectives on Listening

Listening is the effort or work of placing the therapist where the patient is ("lives"). The ear of the empathic listener is the organ of receptivity – gratifying and, at times, indulging the patient. Every human being has a preferred interpersonal stance, a set of relationships and transactions with which she or he is most comfortable and feels most gratified. The problem is that for most psychiatric patients, they do not work well, but the psychiatrist, through listening and observing, must understand the patient. Beyond attitudes that enable or prevent listening, there is a role for specific knowledge. It is important to achieve the cognitive structure or theoretical framework and use it with rigor and discipline in the service of patients so that psychiatrists can employ more than global "feelings" or "hunches". In striving to grasp the inner experience of any other human being, one must know what it is to be human; one must have an idea of what is inside any person. This provides a framework for understanding what the patient – who would not be a patient if he fully understood what was inside of him – is struggling to communicate. Personality theory is absolutely crucial to this process.

Whether we acknowledge it or not, every one of us has a theory of human personality (in this day and age of porous boundaries between psychology and biology, we should really speak of a psychobiological theory of human experience), which we apply in various situations, social or clinical. These theories become part of the template alluded to earlier, which allows certain words, stories, actions, and cues from the patient to jump out with profound meaning to the psychiatrist. There is no substitute for a thorough knowledge of many theories of human functioning and a well-disciplined synthesis and internal set of rules to decide which theories to use in which situations.

Different theoretical positions offer slightly different and often complementary perspectives on listening (Table 1.4). Each of the great schools of psychotherapy places the psychiatrist in a somewhat different relationship to the patient. This may even be reflected in the physical placement of the therapist in relation to the patient. In a classical psychoanalytic stance, the therapist, traditionally unseen behind the patient, assumes an active, hovering attention. Existential analysts seek to experience the patient's position and place themselves close to and facing the patient. The interpersonal psychiatrist stresses a collaborative dialogue with shared control. One can almost imagine the two side by side as the clinician strives to sense what the storyteller is doing to and with the listener. Interpersonal theory stresses the need for each participant to act within that interpersonal social field.

In the object relations stance, the listener keeps in mind the "other people in the room" with him and the storyteller, that is, the patient's introjects who are constantly part of the internal conversation of the patient and thus influence the dialogue within the therapeutic dyad. In connecting with the patient, the listener is also tuned in to the fact that parts and fragments of him or her are being internalized by the patient.

Table 1.4 Theoretical Perspectives on Listening

Theory	Focus of Attention	Listening Stance
Ego psychology	Stream of associations	Neutral, hovering attention
Object relations	Introjects (internalized images of others within the patient)	Neutral, hovering attention
Interpersonal	What relationship is the patient attempting to construct?	Participant observer
Existential	Feelings, affect	Empathic identification with the patient
Self-psychology	Sense of self from others	Empathic mirroring and affirmation
Patient centered	Content control by patient	Noncontingent positive regard, empathy
Cognitive	Hidden assumptions and distortions	Benign expert
Behavioral	Behavioral contingencies	Benign expert
Family systems	Complex forces maneuvering each member	Neutral intruder who forces imbalance in the system

The listener becomes another person in the room of the patient's life experience, within and outside the therapeutic hour. Cognitive and behavioral psychiatrists are kindly experts, listening attentively and subtly for hidden assumptions, distortions, and connections. The family systems psychiatrist sits midway among the pressures and forces emanating from each individual, seeking to affect the system so that all must adapt differently.

Referring again to Clinical Vignette 3, we can see the different theoretical models of the listening process in the discovery of the meaning of "little fella". Freud's model is one in which the psychiatrist had listened repeatedly to a specific association and inquired of its meaning. Object relations theorists would note that the clinician had discovered a previously unidentified, powerful introject within the therapeutic dyad. The interpersonal psychiatrist would see the shared exploration of this idiosyncratic manner of describing one's youth; the patient had been continually trying to take the therapist to "The Andy Griffith Show". That is, the patient was attempting to induce the clinician to share the experience of imagining and fantasizing about having Andy Griffith as a father.

Existentialists would note how the psychiatrist was changed dramatically by the patient's repeated use of this phrase and then altered even more profoundly by the memory of Andy Griffith, "the consummate good father" in the patient's words. The therapist could never see the patient in quite the same way again, and the patient sensed it immediately. And Kohut would note the mirroring quality of the psychiatrist's interpretation of the meaning of this important memory. This would be mirroring at its most powerful, affirming the patient's important differences from his family, helping him to consolidate the memories. The behavioral psychiatrist would note the reciprocal inhibition that had gone on, with Andy Griffith soothing the phobic anxieties in a brutal family.

A cognitive psychiatrist would wonder whether the patient's depression resulted from a hidden assumption that anything less than the idyllic images of television was not good enough. The family systems psychiatrist would help the patient see that he had manipulated the forces at work on him and actually changed the definition of his family.

The ways and tools of listening also change, according to the purpose, the nature of the therapeutic dyad. The ways of listening also change depending upon whether or not the psychiatrist is preoccupied or inattentive. The medical model psychiatrist listens for signs and symptoms. The analyst listens for the truth often clothed in fantasy and metaphor. The existentialist listens for feeling, and the interpersonal theorist listens for the shared experiences engendered by the interaction. Regardless of the theoretical stance and regardless of the mental tension between the medical model's need to know symptoms and signs and the humanistic psychiatrist's listening to know the sufferer, the essence of therapeutic listening is the suspension of judgment before any presentation of the story and the storyteller. The listener is asked to clarify and classify the inner world of the storyteller at the same time he or she is experiencing it – no small feat!

Using Oneself in Listening

Understanding transference and countertransference is crucial to effective listening. Tomkins, LeDoux, Damasio, and Brothers have given us a basic biological perspective on this process. However, one defines these terms, whatever one's theoretical stance about these issues. To know ourselves is to begin to know our patients more deeply. There are many ways to achieve this. Personal therapy is one. Ongoing life experience is another. Supervision that emphasizes one's emotional reactions to patients is still a third. Once we have started on the road to achieving this understanding by therapy, supervision, or life experience, continued listening to our patients, who teach us about ourselves and others, becomes a lifelong method of growth.

To know oneself is to be aware that there are certain common human needs, wishes, fears, feelings, and reactions. Every person must deal in some way with attachment, dependence, authority, autonomy, selfhood, values and ideals, remembered others, work, love, hate, and loss. It is unlikely that the psychiatrist can comprehend the patient without his or her own self-awareness. Thus, Figure 1.1 should really look like Figure 1.2. The most psychotic patient in the world is still struggling with these universal human functions (Clinical Vignette 10).

In this case, the psychiatrist was able to connect with a patient's inner experience in a manner that had a fairly dramatic impact on the clinical course. That is the goal of listening. The art is hearing the patient's inner experience and then addressing it empathically, enabling the patient to feel heard and affirmed. There are no rules about this, and at any given point in a clinical encounter, there are many ways to accomplish it. There are also many ways to respond that are unhelpful and even retraumatizing. The skilled psychiatrist, just as she or he never forgets that it is the patient's inner experience that is to be heard, also never stops struggling to find just the right words, gestures, expressions, and inflections

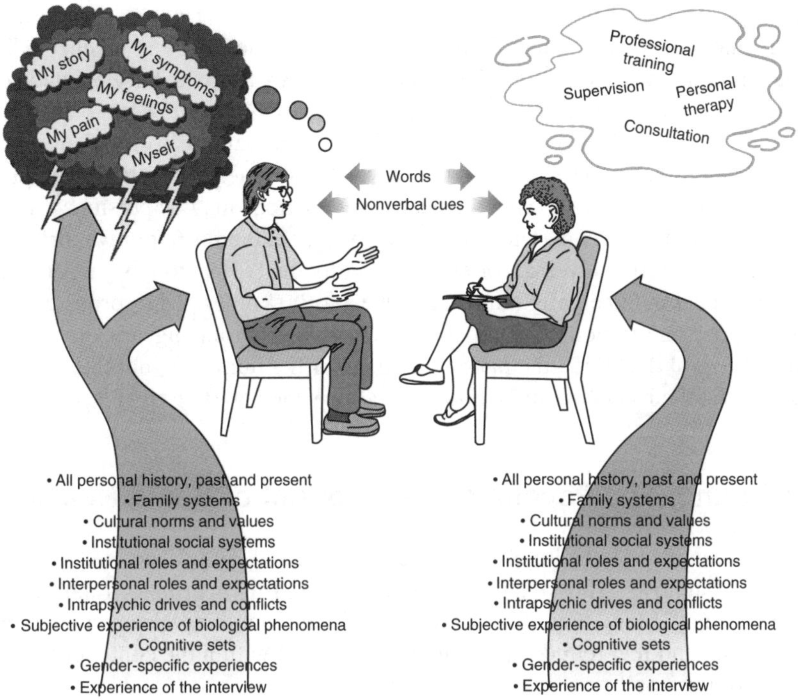
My story
My symptoms
My feelings
My pain
Myself
Professional training
Supervision
Personal therapy
Consultation
Words
Nonverbal cues
• All personal history, past and present
• Family systems
• Cultural norms and values
• Institutional social systems
• Institutional roles and expectations
• Interpersonal roles and expectations
• Intrapsychic drives and conflicts
• Subjective experience of biological phenomena
• Cognitive sets
• Gender-specific experiences
• Experience of the interview
• All personal history, past and present
• Family systems
• Cultural norms and values
• Institutional social systems
• Institutional roles and expectations
• Interpersonal roles and expectations
• Intrapsychic drives and conflicts
• Subjective experience of biological phenomena
• Cognitive sets
• Gender-specific experiences
• Experience of the interview

Figure 1.2 *The therapeutic dyad (Kay and Tasman, 2006).*

Clinical Vignette 10

A young man with paranoid schizophrenia had been admitted in 1979 to the hospital following a near lethal attack on his father. When asked about this incident, he became frankly delusional, speaking of the Arab–Israeli conflict, the preciousness of Jerusalem, how the Israelis must defend it at all costs. Unspoken was his conviction that he was like the Israelis, with the entire world attacking and threatening him. He believed his father had threatened and attacked him when, in fact, his father had done little more than seek to be closer, more comforting, and advising with the patient. The psychiatrist understood the patient to be speaking of that core of selfhood that we all possess, which, when threatened, creates a sense of vulnerability and panic, a disintegrating anxiety unlike any other. The psychiatrist spoke to the patient of Anwar Sadat's visit to Jerusalem and engaged him in a discussion of how that had gone, what the outcome had been, had the threat been lessened or increased? The patient, although still delusional, visibly relaxed and began to speak much more directly about his own sense of vulnerability and uncertainty over his personal integrity and its ability to withstand any closeness. He still required neuroleptic medication for his illness; however, his violent thoughts and behaviors reduced dramatically. He was able to begin interacting with his father, and his behavior on the ward changed as well.

that say to a patient, "you have been understood". The most clever diagnostician or insightful interpreter who cannot "connect" with the patient in this manner will miss valuable information. This issue has been addressed by writers who have pointed out how little understood are the concepts of support and empathy (Peteet, 1982).

Being human is also to be a creature of habit and pattern in linguistic, interpersonal, and emotional realms. The skilled psychiatrist listens with this ever in mind. What we see in the interview, what we hear in interactions may be presumed to be repetitions of many other events. The content may vary, but the form, motive, process, and evolution are generally universal for any given individual. This, too, is part of listening. To know what is fundamentally human, to have a well-synthesized rigorous theory, and to hear the person's unique but repetitive ways of experiencing are the essence of listening. These skills "find" the patient in all his or her humanity, but then the psychiatrist must find the right communication that allows the patient to feel "found".

To Be Found: The Psychological Product of Being Heard

Psychiatric patients may be lonely, isolated, demoralized, and desperate, regardless of the specific diagnosis. They have lost themselves and their primary relationships, if they ever had any. Many therapists believe that before anything else can happen, they must be found, and feel found. They can only be found within the context of their own specific histories, cultures, religions, genders, social contexts, and so on. There is nothing more healing than the experience of being found by another. The earliest expression of this need is in infancy and we refer to it as the need for attachment. Referring to middle childhood, Harry Stack Sullivan spoke of the importance of the pal or buddy. Kohut spoke of the lifelong need for self-objects. In lay terms, it is often subsumed under the need for love, security, and acceptance. Psychiatric patients have lost or never had this experience. However obnoxious or destructive or desperate their overt behavior, it is the psychiatrist's job to seek and find the patient. That is the purpose of listening.

If we look back to Clinical Vignette 3, wherein the phrase "little fella" bespoke such deep and important unverbalized meaning, the patient's reaction to the memory and recognition by the psychiatrist was dramatic. He had always known he was different in some indefinable ways from his family. That difference had been both a source of pride and pain to him at various developmental stages. However, the recognition of the specific source, its meaning, and its constant presence in his life created a whole new sense of himself. He had been found by his psychiatrist, who echoed the discovery, and he had found an entire piece of himself that he had enacted for years, yet which had been disconnected from any integrated sense of himself.

Sometimes objectifying and defining the disease/disorder enables the person to feel found. One of the most challenging patients to hear and experience is the acting out, self-destructive, demanding person with borderline personality disorder. Even as the prior sentence conveys, psychiatrists often experience the diagnosis as who the patient is rather than what he or she suffers. The following case conveys how one third-year resident was able to hear such a patient, and in his listening to her introduce the idea that the symptoms were not her but her disorder (Clinical Vignette 11).

Clinical Vignette 11

The psychiatrist was working the midnight Friday to 11 a.m. Saturday shift in a Psychiatric Emergency Room. The patient was a 26-year-old woman brought in by ambulance after overdosing on sertraline following an argument with her boyfriend. She had been partying with him and became enraged at the attention he was paying to the date of a friend who was accompanying them. After being cleared medically, the patient was transferred to psychiatry for crisis intervention. It was about 4 a.m. when she arrived. She was crying and screaming for the psychiatric staff to release her. In the emergency department, she had grabbed a suture scissors attached to the uniform of the charge nurse. The report was given to the psychiatric resident that she had been a "management problem" in the medicine ER.

The psychiatrist sat wearily and listened to the patient tell her story with tears, shouts, and expletives sputtered through clenched teeth. She stated that she did not remember ever being happy, that she frequently had thoughts of suicide, and that she had overdosed twice before, following a divorce from her first husband at the age of 19 and then 8 months prior to this episode when she had been fired from a job for arguing with her supervisor. Her parents had kept her 6-year-old and 7-year-old sons since her divorce. She was currently working as a file clerk and living with her boyfriend of 2 months. She stated that she felt like there was a cold ice cube stuck in her chest as she watched her boyfriend flirting with the other woman. She acknowledged that she felt empty and utterly alone even in the crowded bar. She created an unpleasant scene and they continued to argue until they got home. Then he had laughed at her and left, stating that he would come back when she had cooled down.

The resident sat quietly and listened. He looked dreary. The night had been a busy one. She looked at him and complained, "Don't let me and my problems bore you!" He looked at her and said, "Quite the contrary. I've been thinking as you speak that I know what disorder you suffer from". With that statement, he pulled out the DSM-IV and read with her the description of the symptoms and signs of borderline personality disorder. She had been in therapy off and on since she was 16 years old. No one had ever shared with her the name of the diagnosis but instead had responded to her as if the disorder was the definition of who she was. In his listening, he was able to hear her symptoms as a disorder and not the person. And in his ability to separate the two, he was able to allow her to distance herself from the symptoms, too, and see herself in a new light with her first inkling of her own personhood.

Gender can play a significant role in the experience of feeling found. Some individuals feel that it is easier to connect with a person of the same sex; others, with someone of the opposite sex. Clinical Vignette 6 is an excellent example of this. In these days of significant change in and sensitivity to sex roles, a misinterpretation such as that early in treatment could result in a permanent rupture in the alliance. Psychiatrists vary in their sensitivity to

Table 1.5 The Basic Sciences of Listening
Neurobiology of primary affects
Universality of certain affective expressions
Neurobiology of empathy
Biological need for interpersonal regulation
Psychobiology of attachment
Biological impact of social support
Environmental impact on central nervous system structure and function

the different sexes. Some may do better with those who have chosen more traditional roles; others may be more sensitive to those who have adopted more modern roles.

We now know that just as there is a neurobiological basis for empathy and countertransference, there is a similar biological basis for the power of listening to heal, to lift psychological burdens, to remoralize, and to provide emotional regulation to patients who feel out of control in their rage, despair, terror, or other feelings (Table 1.5). Attachment and social support are psychobiological processes that provide the necessary physiological regulation to human beings. A neurobiological view supports the notion of the patient's capacity to perceive empathy through the powerful nonverbal, universally understood communication of facial expressions. His research in basic human emotions sets forth the idea of their understanding across cultures and ages. It further supports the provocative idea that facial expressions of the listener may generate autonomic and central nervous system changes not only within the listener but within the one being heard, and vice versa. Indeed, the evidence is growing that new experiences in clinical interactions create learning and new memories, which are associated with changes in both brain structure and function. When we listen in this way, we are intervening not only in a psychological manner to connect, heal, and share burdens but also in a neurobiological fashion to regulate, modulate, and restore functioning. When patients feel found, they are responding to this psychobiological process.

Listening to Oneself to Listen Better

To hold in mind what has been said and heard after a session and between sessions is the most powerful and active tool of listening. It is a crucial step often overlooked by students and those new at listening. It is necessary to hear our patients in our thoughts during the in-between times in order to pull together repetitive patterns of thinking, behaving, and feeling, giving us the closest idea of how patients experience themselves and their world. In addition, many of our traumatized patients have not had the experience of being held in mind, of being remembered, and their needs being thought of by significant others. These key experiences of childhood affirm the young person's psychological being. It is important to distinguish this kind of "re-listening" to the patient – an important part of the psychiatrist's ongoing processing and reprocessing of what has been heard and experienced – from what some may leap to call countertransference. One way of identifying this distinction would be to differentiate listening to oneself as one reviews in one's mind the patient's story versus becoming preoccupied and stuck with one's thoughts and feelings about a particular aspect of a patient (Clinical Vignette 12).

As the verbal interaction with the patient occurs, psychiatrists may find themselves expressing thoughts and feeling in ways that may be quite different from their usual repertoire. The following case is an example.

This sort of listening to oneself in order to understand the patient requires a good working knowledge of projective identification. Projective identification is a phrase

Clinical Vignette 12

A second-year resident, rotating through an inpatient unit that serves the psychiatric needs of very severely ill psychotic patients with multiple admissions, dual diagnoses, homelessness, criminal records, significant histories of medical noncompliance, and, in some, unremitting psychosis, was particularly struggling with a 33-year-old white woman admitted for the 11th time since age 19. The patient invariably stopped medications shortly after discharge, never kept follow-up appointments, and ended up on the streets psychotic and high on crack cocaine. She would then be involuntarily committed for restabilization. And so the cycle would repeat itself. The resident would see the patient on daily rounds. The patient's litany was the same day after day: "I'm not sick. I don't need to be here. I don't need medicines". And regularly she refused doses.

The resident spoke often of her patient to other residents in her class and often found herself ruminating about the patient's abject lostness. She began her regular supervision hours either frustrated or feeling hopeless that anything would change with this patient because the patient flatly refused to acknowledge her disorder. The patient's level of denial was of psychotic proportions. Shortly after a particularly difficult encounter with the patient concerning her refusal to take an evening dose of haloperidol, the resident came to supervision with the report that she had awakened terrorized by dreaming the night before that she had been diagnosed with schizophrenia. She had been intensely affected by overwhelming pain, confusion, and despair as she heard the diagnosis in her dream. "IT CAN'T BE!" she screamed, waking herself with a shaking start. "I'M NOT SICK! I DON'T NEED TO BE HERE! I DON'T NEED MEDICINE!" The words of her patient echoed in her mind as her own echoed in her ears. She had taken the patient's story and words home with her and kept them in mind at an unconscious level to be brought up in her dream, the ultimate identification with the patient. How more intensely can one be empathic with her patient than to dream as if she is experiencing the same horrifying reality? The patient and resident continued to struggle, but after the dream the resident was able to approach the patient and her story from a position of understanding the patient's need to maintain a lack of awareness or absence of insight. To acknowledge the presence of the disorder was more than the patient's already fragmented ego could bear. And now the resident "heard" it.

used to describe a defense mechanism in which the patient, in an effort to master intolerably terrifying emotions, unconsciously seeks to engender them in the therapist and to identify with the psychiatrist's ability to tolerate and handle the feelings (Clinical Vignettes 13 and 14).

Clinical Vignette 13

A 45-year-old divorced white woman, being followed for bipolar disorder and borderline personality traits and stable for several years on lithium, was in weekly psychotherapy. During the prior weekend, she had moved into another apartment closer to her work. On the day of the move, she overslept and woke up with a start. The admonition to herself as she awoke was, "You lazy bitch! You can never manage on your own". She had earlier, as a child, experienced a mother who was needy, engulfing, punishing, hostile, critical, and dependent upon the patient. Her therapist, having some knowledge of the patient and her background, said, "Your mother is still with you. It was she in your head continuing to bombard you with derogatory statements". The same patient was often 10 or 15 minutes late for sessions, and her therapist found herself irritated at the patient's habitual tardiness. To her own surprise and enlightenment, the therapist also found herself thinking, "What a chaotic woman! She'll never manage to be here on time". She, too, had heard the voice of her patient's mother. In the next session, she wondered with her patient if she found herself wishing to place her therapist in the position of her mother, wanting at once to be engulfed and punished.

Clinical Vignette 14

A psychiatrist was treating a 40-year-old man who was in the process of recognizing his own primary homosexual orientation. In the course of treatment, he became enraged, suicidal, and homicidal. After one session, the psychiatrist, while driving home, experienced the fantasy that when he got home, he would find his patient already there, having taken the psychiatrist's family hostage. The psychiatrist became increasingly terrified, even outright paranoid that this fantasy might actually come to pass. The patient was a computer expert who had indeed discovered the unlisted phone number and address of his therapist. But the psychiatrist realized that this fantasy was far out of keeping with his own usual way of feeling and the patient's way of behaving and viewing him. On arriving home to discover his family quite safe, the psychiatrist called the patient and scheduled him as his first for appointment the following morning. When the patient arrived, the psychiatrist said, "You know, I think I'm only now beginning to appreciate just how terrified and desperate all of this makes you". The patient slumped down into his chair, heaved a sigh, and said, "Thank God!"

Listening in Special Clinical Situations

Children

Listening to younger children often involves inviting them to play and then engaging them in describing what is happening in the play action. The psychiatrist pays careful attention to the child's feelings. These feelings are usually attributed to a doll, puppet, or other humanized toy. So if a child describes a stuffed animal as being scared, the psychiatrist may say, "I wonder if you, too, are scared when…" or "That sounds like you when…". The following case is an example (Clinical Vignette 15).

Clinical Vignette 15

A 4-year-old boy was brought in for psychiatric evaluation. He and his father had come upon a very serious automobile accident. One person had been thrown from the car and was lying clearly visible on the pavement with arms and legs positioned in grotesque angles, gaping head wound, obviously dead. The child's father was an off-duty police officer who stopped to assist in the extraction of two other people trapped in the car. The father kept a careful eye on the youngster who was left in the car. The child observed the scene for about 30 minutes until others arrived on the scene and his dad was able to leave. That night and for days to come, the child preoccupied himself with his toy cars, which he repetitiously rammed into each other. He was awakened by nightmares three times in the ensuing weeks. During his evaluation in the play therapy room, he engaged in ramming toy cars together. In addition, he tossed dolls about and arranged their limbs haphazardly. As he was encouraged to put some words to his action, he spoke of being frightened of the dead body and of being afraid to be by himself. He was afraid of the possibility of being hurt himself. He came in for three more play sessions, which went much the same way. His preoccupation with ramming cars at home diminished and disappeared as did the nightmares. The content of his play was used to help him put words and labels on his scare.

Geriatric Patients

Working with the elderly poses its own special challenges. These challenges include not only the unique developmental issues they face but also the difficulty in verbalizing a lifetime of experience and feelings, and, commonly, a disparity in age and life experience between the clinician and the patient.

It is challenging to elicit the elements of a story, especially when they span generations. The elderly are often stoic. In the face of losses that mark the closing years of life, denial often becomes a healthy tool, allowing one to accept and cope with declining abilities and the loss of loved ones. The psychiatrist must appreciate that grief and depression can often be similar in some respects (Clinical Vignette 16).

Clinical Vignette 16

A psychiatrist was asked to examine an 87-year-old white man whom the family believed to be depressed. They stated that he was becoming increasingly detached and disinterested in the goings-on around him. When seen, he was cooperative and compliant, but he stated that he didn't believe he needed to be evaluated. The patient had faced multiple losses over the past few years. After retiring at the age of 65, he had developed the habit of meeting male friends at a coffee shop each morning at 7 a.m. Now, all but he and one other were dead, and the other was in a nursing home with the cognitive deficits of primary dementia of the Alzheimer's type, preventing his friend from recognizing him when visiting. The patient's wife had died 15 years ago after many years of marriage. He had missed her terribly at first but then after a year or so he got on with his life. Several years later, he suffered a retinal detachment that impaired his vision to the point that he was no longer able to drive himself to get about as he once had. What he missed most was the independence of going places when it suited him, rather than relying on his son or grandson to accommodate him within their busy schedules. He had taken to watching televised church services rather than trouble his son to drive him to church. His mind remained sharp, he said, but his body was wearing out, and all the people with whom he had shared a common history had died. His answers were "fine" and "all right" when questions of quality of sleep and mood were asked – despite the fact that he had experienced significant nocturia. When questioned about his ability to experience joy, he retorted, "Would you be?" His youngest sister had died the year prior to the evaluation. She was 76 years old and had been on home oxygen for the last 18 months of her life for end-stage chronic obstructive pulmonary disease. He had been particularly close to her because she was only 3 years old when their mother had died. He had been her caretaker all her life.

Although he denied feelings of guilt, he said that it "wasn't right" that he had outlived the youngest member of his family. His family said that he had taken her death especially hard and was tearful and angry. The focus of his anger during the final stages of her illness was at the young doctors whom he perceived as having given up on her. After her death, it fell to him to dispose of her accumulated possessions as she had no children and her husband had preceded her in death many years before. At first, he said that he couldn't face the task. Finally, some 2 months later, he was able to close her estate. During that period of time, he had significant sleep disturbance, reduced energy, and his family often experienced him as crotchety and complaining. They and the patient attributed it to mourning her loss. However, recently he was emotionally detached, not very interested in life around him, and they found it particularly alarming that he had said to his son that he was "ready to die". What did all this mean? Was he depressed? Was he physically ill, creating the sense of apathy and disinterest? Was he grieving? He was not suicidal. He did not suffer negative thoughts about his own personhood. He was not having thoughts that he had let anyone down. Together, he and the psychiatrist decided that he was indeed grieving. This time, he was grieving for his own decline and imminent death. He, in fact, was in the final acceptance phase of that process. In a family meeting, in the discussions about the feelings of each member of the family, it became apparent that he was facing the end of life, which evoked many emotions in those who loved him.

Chronically Mentally Ill

Listening to the chronically mentally ill can be especially challenging, too. The unique choice of words characteristic of many who have a thought disorder requires that the physician search for the meanings of certain words and phrases that may be peculiar and truly eccentric. Clinical Vignettes 1, 10, and 12 are examples of this important challenge for the psychiatric listener (Clinical Vignettes 17 and 18).

Clinical Vignette 17

A young man with schizotypal personality disorder and obsessive–compulsive disorder presented for months using adjectives describing himself as "broken and fragmented". Only after listening carefully, not aided by the expected or normal affect of a depressed person, was the psychiatrist able to discern that his patient was clinically depressed but did not have the usual words to say it or was unable to discuss it.

Clinical Vignette 18

A 32-year-old black woman who had multiple hospitalizations for schizophrenia and lived with her mother was seen in the community psychiatric center for routine medication follow-up. Her psychiatrist found her to have an increase in the frequency of auditory hallucinations, especially ones of a derogatory nature. The voices were tormenting her with the ideas that she was not good, that she should die, that she was worthless and unloved. Her psychiatrist heard her say that she had wrecked her mother's car 2 weeks previously. The streets had been wet and the tires worn. She had slid into the rear of a car that had come to an abrupt stop ahead of her on a freeway. Although her mother had not been critical or judgmental, the patient felt overwhelming guilt as she watched her mother struggle to arrange transportation for herself each day to and from work.

Chronically psychiatrically disabled patients may have a unique way of presenting their inner world experiences. Sometimes the link to the outer world is not so apparent. The psychiatrist is regularly challenged with making sense of the meanings of the content and changes in intensity or frequency of the psychotic symptoms.

Physically Ill Patients

In consultations with a colleague in a medical or surgical specialty, one is evaluating a patient who has a chronic or acute physical illness. The psychiatrist must listen to the story of the patient but also keep in mind the story as reflected in the hospital records and medical and nursing staff. Then the psychiatrist serves as the liaison not only between psychiatry and other medical colleagues, but also between the patient and his or her caregivers (Clinical Vignette 19).

Clinical Vignette 19

A 35-year-old woman was hospitalized for complications of a pancreas/kidney transplant that was completed 20 months previously. Prior to surgery she had been on dialysis for over a year awaiting a tissue match for transplantation. That year she had been forced to take a leave of absence from her job as a social worker with a local child and adolescent community center. At the time of this hospitalization, she had been back at work for only 8 months when she developed a urinary tract infection that did not respond to several antibiotics. Her renal function was deteriorating and her doctors found her to be paranoid, hostile, and labile. Her physicians dreaded going into her room each morning and began distancing themselves from her.

Psychiatric consultation was sought following a particularly difficult interaction between the patient and her charge nurse, the leader of the transplant team, and the infectious disease expert. She was hostile, blaming, agitated, circumstantial, refused further medications, and pulled out her intravenous lines. The consultation requested assistance in hospital management.

When interviewed, the patient was lying quietly in bed but visibly stiffened when the psychiatrist introduced herself. She very quickly exhibited the symptoms described in the consultation. This patient had struggled with juvenile onset diabetes since the age of 9. Despite the fact that she consistently complied with diet and insulin, control of blood sugars had always been difficult. As complication after complication occurred, she often developed the belief that her physicians thought that she was a "bad" patient. And now, the hope that her life would normalize to the point that she could carry on with her career was dashed. She felt misunderstood and alone in her struggle with long-term, chronic illness. The psychiatrist resonated with the story emotionally and listened for ways to address symptoms from a biological standpoint as well. The patient felt reassured that someone was there to appreciate the tragic turn that her life had taken.

Growing and Maturing as a Listener

Transference/countertransference influences not only relationships in traditional psychotherapy but also interactions between all physicians and patients and is always present as a filter or reverberator to that which is heard. However, even the most experienced of listeners are not always aware of the ways in which their patients' stories are impacted by countertransference. Patients come, too, with tendencies and predispositions to experience the listener, the other person in the therapeutic dyad, in familiar but distorted fashion. The patient may idealize and adapt to interpretations. She or he may be hostile and distrustful, identifying the psychiatrist in an unconscious way with one who has been rejecting in the past. Listening to the "flow of consciousness", the psychiatrist discerns a thread of continuity and purposefulness in the patient's communications. As the psychiatrist becomes more and more familiar with his or her patient, he or she will discover the connections between threads and the meaning will become apparent. This awareness may come as a sign and symptom, fantasy, feeling, or fact.

There is an increasing recognition that to be a healing listener one must be able to bear the burden of hearing what is told. Like the patient, we fear what might be said. A patient's story may be one of rage in response to early childhood attachment ruptures or abuse, of sadness as losses are remembered, or of terror in response to disorganization during the experience of perceptual abnormalities accompanying psychotic breaks. The patient's stories invariably invoke anger, shame, guilt, abject helplessness, or sexual feelings within the listener. These feelings, unless attended to, appreciated, and understood, will block the listening that is essential for healing to take place. Every insight is colored by what the listener has known. It is impossible to know that which is not experienced. The psychiatrist comes with his or her own experiences and the experiences he or she has had with others. To listen in the manner we are describing here is another way of truly experiencing the world. The experiences include the imaginings of how it must be to be 87 years old as a patient when one is a 35-year-old doctor just finishing residency, to be female when one is male, to be a child again, to grow up African-American in a small white suburb of a large city, to be an immigrant in a new country, to be Middle Eastern when one is Western European, and so on. One comes to know by listening with imagination, allowing the words of the patient to resonate with one's own experiences or with what one has come to know through hearing with imagination the stories of other patients or listening to the thoughts or insights of supervisors (Clinical Vignette 20).

Clinical Vignette 20

A Jewish resident was treating an 8-year-old Catholic boy who came in one day and mentioned offhandedly that he was about to go to his first confession. The psychiatric resident made no particular note of the issue and kept on listening to the boy's play and its themes. He noted that guilt, which had been an ongoing theme, was prominent again. When he presented the session in supervision, the supervisor wondered about the connection. It emerged that there was a large gulf between the therapist and the boy. Jewish concepts of sin and atonement are different from Christian ones, and the rituals surrounding them have rather different intentions and ideas of resolution. The resident had missed the opportunity to explore the young boy's first introduction, within his religious context, to the belief in a forgiving God, a potentially important step in helping the child to resolve his ongoing struggles with guilt over his own greedy impulses.

The best psychiatrists continue all their professional lives to learn how to listen better. This may be thought of not only as a matter of mastering countertransference but of self-education. One must learn to recognize when there are impasses in the treatment and to seek education, from a colleague or, perhaps, even from the patient. Consider these two examples.

How can the psychiatrist's demeanor convey to the patient that he or she is safe to tell his or her story, that the listener is one who can be trusted to be with him or her, to worry with him or her, and serve as a helper? Much is written about the demeanor of the psychiatrist. The air, deportment, manner, or bearing is one of quiet anticipation – to receive that which the patient has come to tell and share in the telling. Signals of anticipation and curiosity may be conveyed by such statements as "I've thought about what you said last time", "How do you feel about…?", "What if…?" (Clinical Vignette 21).

Clinical Vignette 21

A psychiatrist began treating a Nigerian native who was suffering from posttraumatic stress disorder (PTSD) after being assaulted at work. After several sessions, the psychiatrist felt a sense of being at a loss in terms of what the patient was expecting out of their work and how the therapist was being seen by the patient. He then took several sessions to inquire of the patient about his tribe, its structure, family roles, definitions of healing, ideas of illness and wellness, etc. After this exploration, the psychiatrist adopted a different stance with the patient, heard the patient's communications very differently, and the therapy proceeded much more smoothly and comfortably to a successful conclusion.

Efforts of clarification often serve as bridges between sessions and communicate that the listener is committed to a fuller understanding of the patient. Patients have the need to experience the psychiatrist as empathic. Empathy describes the feeling one has in hearing a story which causes one to conjure up or imagine how it would have been to have actually have had an experience oneself. How does one integrate all this so that it is automatic but not deadened by automaticity? How does the psychiatrist continue to hear the "same old thing" with freshness and renewal? How does one encourage the patient with consistency, clarity, and assurance in the face of uncertainty and occasional confusion? Not by assurance that everything will be all right when things might probably not be. Not by attempting to talk the patient into seeing things the clinician's way but rather by the psychiatrist's having the capacity to hear things his or her patient's way, from the patient's perspective.

Psychiatry is one of those rare disciplines where the experience of listening over and over again allows the listener to grow in their capacities to hear and to heal. Hopefully, we get better and better as the years advance, become smoother, and develop a style that blends with our personality and training. We are renewed by the shared experiences with our patients.

To hear stories of the human condition reminds the psychiatrist that he or she, too, is human. There is time to make discoveries in the patient's stories from previous times, and maybe in previous patients. Patients will always endeavor to tell their stories. The psychiatrist continues to grow by being the perpetual student, always with an ear for the lesson, the remarkable life stories of his or her patients.

References

Binswanger L (1963) *Being in the World*. Basic Books, New York.

Elkin I, Shea MT, Watkins JT *et al*. (1989) National Institute of Mental Health Treatment of Depression Collaborative Research Program: General effectiveness of treatments. *Archives of General Psychiatry* 46(11), 971–982.

Kay J and Tasman A (2006) *Essentials of Psychiatry*. John Wiley & Sons, Inc., Hoboken.

Peteet JR (1982) A closer look at the concept of support: Some application to the care of patients with cancer. *General Hospital Psychiatry* 4(1), 19–23.

Schore AN (2001) The effects of a secure attachment relationship: Right brain development, affect regulation, and infant mental health. *Infant Mental Health Journal* 22, 7–66.

CHAPTER

2 Physician–Patient Relationship

For centuries, healers had little understanding of disease and lacked the technologies we now know are necessary for the treatment and cure of many diseases. Physicians had few medications, and surgery was only a last resort. In fact, the most important tool for healing was the relationship between the physician and the patient. It is well known that social connectedness enhances health in both direct and indirect ways: directly regulating many biological functions, decreasing anxiety, providing opportunities for new information, and fostering alternative behaviors. Clinical wisdom holds that both the reality-based elements of the physician–patient relationship – in modern times referred to as the working alliance or the therapeutic alliance – and the fantasy-based elements of that relationship affect the patient's pain, suffering, and recovery from illness.

Historically, often the physician's only interventions were reassuring patients, providing knowledge about the patient's disease, accepting the patient's feelings of distress as normal, and maximizing the patient's hope for the future. Although these interventions, based on wisdom and intuition, are no longer the only tools available to the physician, they continue to be an important part of the physician's and particularly the psychiatrist's therapeutic armamentarium.

Such nonspecific aspects of cure are often thought to be mystical or mysterious. In fact, in biological studies, they are recognized as the placebo effect. Oddly, these effects of interpersonal relationships are both one of the prized and one of the most denigrated aspects of all of medicine. Yet, as clinicians, we all strive to alleviate our patients' pain and suffering and return them to health as soon as possible with whatever tools may help. Many well-designed studies show that 20–30% of subjects respond to the placebo condition. Recent studies show that analgesic placebo has similar neural mechanisms to opioid analgesia (Petrovic *et al.*, 2002). The problem with placebos is not whether they work but that we do not understand how they work and, therefore, we do not have control over their effects. As a physician, one strives to maximize one's interpersonal healing effects and, in this way as well as with other healing tools, increase the chances of our patients' relief from pain and of recovery.

The physician–patient relationship includes specific roles and motivations. These form the core ingredients of the healing process. In its most generic form, the physician–patient

The Psychiatric Interview: Evaluation and Diagnosis, First Edition. Allan Tasman, Jerald Kay and Robert J. Ursano.

This chapter is based on Chapter 2 (Amy M. Ursano, Stephen M. Sonnenberg, Robert J. Ursano) of *Psychiatry*, 3rd Edition.

relationship is defined by the coming together of an expert and a help seeker to identify, understand, and solve the problems of the help seeker. The patient is motivated by the desire and hope for assistance and relief from pain, and the physician has an interest in people and a desire to help. Caring about and paying attention to a patient's suffering can yield remarkable therapeutic dividends. More than one attending physician has been reminded of this when a patient deferred making a treatment decision until he or she was able to consult with "my doctor", who turned out to be the medical student.

In today's technology-driven medicine, the importance and complexity of the physician–patient interaction are often overlooked. The amount of information the medical student or resident must learn frequently takes precedence over learning the fine points of helping the patient relax sufficiently to provide a thorough history or to allow the physician to palpate a painful abdomen. Talking with patients and understanding the intricacies of the physician–patient relationship may be given little formal attention in the medical school curriculum. Even so, medical students, residents, and staff physicians recognize, often with awe, the skill of the senior physician who uncovers the lost piece of history, motivates the patient who had given up hope, or is able to talk to the distressed family without increasing their sense of hopelessness or fear.

The relationship between the physician and the patient is essential to the healing of many patients, perhaps particularly so for many psychiatric patients. The physician who can skillfully recognize the patient's half-hidden comment that he or she has not been taking the prescribed medication, perhaps hidden because of feelings of shame, anger, or denial, is better able to ensure long-term compliance with medication as well as to motivate the patient to stay in treatment. Regardless of the type of treatment – medication, biofeedback, hospitalization, psychotherapy, or the rearrangement of the demands and responsibilities in the patient's life – the relationship with the physician is critical to therapeutic outcome.

Modern medicine emphasizes a specific role for the physician in the relationship with the patient. In many Western countries, the patient comes for help with a specific problem, and the doctor's office staff secures permission from a third-party payer for the doctor to conduct a particular treatment, a prescribed intervention, which will take a specified amount of time. Decades ago, when the doctor was neighbor, advisor, and friend to the patient and routinely invited to important family events in the patient's life such as weddings of children, and when doctors routinely cared for more than one generation of the same family, the physician typically assumed that he or she would be a source of strength and assistance to the patient throughout the cycle of life. This meant more than curing a specific disease or relieving a specific pain.

While today's patients may not consciously expect that the physician's influence and healing powers will take many forms in a complex interpersonal relationship, human nature is still the same, and patients still want from their doctors many nonspecific forms of emotional support that can promote a sense of well-being and better health. Though modern doctors may feel a great deal of time pressure to see many patients each day and to focus narrowly their healing efforts, the physician must also be sensitive to the many needs of patients, who believe that the physician is possessed of wisdom and understanding. Sensitivity to such desires and needs will promote effective medical care in all specialties, with all patients. A view that such patients are unusually needy and demanding will not serve the cause of effective medical care.

Finally, in today's mobile and geographically evermore united world, the importance of recognizing the needs of patients from parts of the world other than that of the physician's is a challenge to the practitioner. The physician must be open to the limitations of his or her knowledge of the expectations, beliefs, and likely behavior of patients from different cultures, nations, religions, and ethnic and socioeconomic backgrounds. The physician must recognize this challenge and, one hopes, embrace it with enthusiasm. It can make the practice of medicine a more exciting experience (Clinical Vignette 1).

Clinical Vignette 1

A 20-year-old female patient suffered a painful athletic injury. She was unsure exactly how her injury had occurred, but she did recall falling on her shoulder on the tennis court while running after a sharply hit ball. She went to the physician fearing that she had damaged her collarbone. When she was informed that there was no fracture, that her pain was due to a bruised muscle and would go away with ice, heat, and aspirin, she immediately felt better. Not only was she relieved but also her perception and experience of the pain actually changed: "It doesn't seem to hurt as much now".

The physician–patient relationship is also a source of information for the physician. The way the patient relates to the physician can help the physician understand the problems the patient is experiencing in her or his interpersonal relationships. The nature of the physician–patient relationship can also provide information about relationships in the patient's childhood family, in which interpersonal patterns are first learned. With this information, the physician can better understand the patient's experience, promote cooperation between the patient and those who care for her or him, and teach the patient new behavioral strategies in an empathic manner, understanding the patient's subjective perspective, that is, feelings, thoughts, and behaviors.

These clinical vignettes illustrate that the physician–patient relationship is composed of both the reality-based component (the working alliance or therapeutic alliance) and the fantasy-based component (the transference) derived from the patient's patterns of interpersonal behavior learned in childhood. These may maximize or limit the patient's sense of reassurance, available information, feelings of comfort, and sense of hope. In this way, the nonspecific curative aspects of the physician–patient relationship may be enhanced or diminished (Clinical Vignettes 2 and 3).

Clinical Vignette 2

Somewhat different was the situation of a 30-year-old male patient who developed chronic pain after an athletic injury. The patient had to convince himself to visit the physician. He felt he was being a "baby" to complain. One week after the injury, he went to his family physician who perfunctorily prescribed a strong painkiller and offered a follow-up appointment a month later. He left feeling that he had been a nuisance. The following week was a particularly bad one for the patient; the pain was severe. But the patient stopped taking the prescribed medication, did not keep the follow-up appointment, and never returned for help. This patient continued to experience pain, unnecessarily, for years. In large part, this was because the physician offered no hope; therefore, follow-up care, including physical therapy and alternative medications, could not be provided.

Clinical Vignette 3

A 45-year-old single man was hospitalized for treatment of a bleeding ulcer. The patient had no past history of ulcers. Despite reassurance, he continued to feel hopeless. A psychiatric consultant was called to evaluate the patient. She found him to be needy, but could not understand why he was so pessimistic. The psychiatrist recognized how important it was to this patient for her to show interest in him, show concern for his condition, and spend time with him. The patient's response was noteworthy; he clearly enjoyed the psychiatrist's company but seemed unusually sad when their times together ended. The psychiatrist asked the patient if this was a correct perception and, if so, why it was the case. The patient responded that the psychiatrist reminded him of his mother. Further inquiry revealed that the patient's mother had died several years ago of colon cancer. The psychiatrist inquired about the symptoms the mother had during her terminal illness. The symptoms were similar to the patient's symptoms: bleeding in the digestive tract and gastrointestinal pain.

The psychiatrist then understood the complex process through which the patient was feeling inordinately pessimistic. Transference was evident in his experience of each departure as an unconscious reminder of the loss of his mother. The patient's identification with his mother (as part of managing her death) was also the source of his unspoken expectation that he, too, was dying of colon cancer. It was the pattern of the relationship between the psychiatrist and the patient, the sadness shown whenever the psychiatrist left, that provided the information necessary to help the patient. Increasing the patient's understanding of his medical condition, specifically how it was different from his mother's, relieved his emotional pain, and he thus began his road to recovery.

Formation of the Physician–Patient Relationship

Assessment and Evaluation

The physician–patient relationship develops during the assessment and evaluation of the patient. The patient observes the thoroughness and sensitivity with which the physician collects information, performs the physical examination, and explains needed tests. At each step, the physician's clarification of the treatment goals and interventions either builds up the patient's expectation of help and feelings of safety or creates increasing disease for the patient. In many aspects, the physician's compassion and patience establishes the context in which learning and growth may occur and anxiety decrease. Alertness to the patient's fears and misunderstandings of the evaluation process can minimize unnecessary disruptions of the relationship and provide information on the patient's previous experiences with medical care and important authority figures, which influence the patient's present expectations of either help or disappointment (Table 2.1).

Table 2.1	Mechanisms for the Formation of the Physician–Patient Relationship
Assessment and evaluation process	
Development of physician–patient rapport	
Therapeutic or working alliance	
Transference	
Countertransference	
Defense mechanisms	
Patient's mental status	

Rapport

Early in the relationship between a psychiatrist and a patient, the patient requests help with his or her pain, uncertainty, or discomfort. The psychiatrist initiates the "contract" of the relationship by acknowledging the patient's pain and offering help. In this action, the psychiatrist has recognized the patient's ill-health and acknowledged the need for and possibility of removing the disease or illness. In this first stage of the development of rapport, the way of relating between the physician and the patient, the physician–patient relationship has begun to organize the interactions. Through the physician's and the patient's shared recognition of the patient's pain, the basis for rapport – a comfortable pattern of working together – is established.

The psychiatrist's ability to empathize, to understand in feeling terms every patient's subjective experience, is important to the development of rapport. Empathy is particularly important in complex interpersonal behavioral problems in which the environment (family, friends, caretakers) may wish to expel the patient, and the patient has therefore lost hope. Suicidal patients, adolescents involved in intense family conflicts, and patients in conflict with their medical caregivers can often be convinced to cooperate with the evaluation only when the psychiatrist has shown accurate empathy early in the first meeting with the patient. This rapport establishes a set of principles of and expectations for the physician–patient interaction. On this basic building block, more elaborate goals and responsibilities of the patient can be developed (Clinical Vignette 4).

Clinical Vignette 4

A young man sought treatment for ill-defined reasons: he was dissatisfied with his work, his social life, and his relationship with his parents. He was unable to say how he thought the psychiatrist could help him, but he knew he was experiencing emotional pain: he felt sadness, anxiety, inhibition, and loss of a lust for living. He wanted help. The psychiatrist noted the patient's tentative style and heard him describe his ambivalence toward his controlling and directing father. With this in mind, the psychiatrist articulated the patient's wish for help and recognized with him his confusion about what was troubling him. She suggested that through discussion they might define together what he was looking for and how she might help him. This description of the evaluation process as a joint process of discovery established a rapport based on shared work, which removed the patient's fears of control and allowed him to feel heard, supported, and involved in the process of regaining his health.

The Therapeutic or Working Alliance

With more disturbed patients, considerable skill is required of the physician to reach this reality-based part of the patient and decrease the patient's fears and expectations of attack or humiliation. Even for healthy patients, the physician must bridge the gap between the patient and the physician, which is always present because of their different backgrounds and perceptions of the world. This gap is an expectable result of differences between the physician's and the patient's culture, gender, ethnic background, socioeconomic class, religion, age, or role in the physician–patient relationship. The experienced physician makes communication across the gap seem effortless, using a different "language" for each patient. The student often sees this as an art rather than as a skill to be learned.

The therapeutic alliance is extremely important in times of crisis such as suicidality, hospitalization, and aggressive behavior. But it is also the basis of agreement about appointments, fees, and treatment requirements. In psychiatric patients, this core component of the physician–patient relationship can be disturbed and requires careful tending. Frequently, the psychiatrist may feel that he or she is "threading a needle" to reach and maintain the therapeutic alliance while not activating the more disturbed elements of the patient's patterns of interpersonal relating.

The therapeutic or working alliance must endure in spite of what may, at times, be intense, irrational, delusional, characterologic, or transference-based feelings of love and hate. The working alliance must outweigh or counterbalance the distorted components of the relationship. It must provide a stable base for the patient and the physician when the patient's feelings or behaviors may impair reflection and cooperation. The working alliance embodies the mutual responsibilities both physician and patient have accepted to restore the patient's health. Likewise, the working alliance must be strong enough to ensure that the treatment goes forward even when both members of the dyad may doubt that it can. The alliance requires a basic trust by the patient that the physician is working in his or her best interests, despite how the patient may feel at a given moment. Patients must be taught to be partners in the healing process and to recognize that the physician is a committed partner in that process as well. The development of common goals fosters the physician and patient seeing themselves as having reciprocal responsibilities: the physician to work in a physician-like fashion to promote healing; the patient to participate actively in formulating and supporting the treatment plan, "trying on" more adaptive behaviors in the chosen mode of treatment, and taking responsibility for his or her actions to the extent possible (Ursano and Silberman, 1988).

Important to the reality-based relationship with the patient is the physician's ability to recognize and acknowledge the limitations of her or his knowledge and to work collaboratively with other physicians. When this happens, patients are most often appreciative, not critical, and experience a strengthening of the alliance because of the physician's commitment to finding an answer. When a patient loses confidence in the physician, it is often because of unacknowledged shortcomings in the physician's skills. The patient may lose motivation to maintain the alliance and seek help elsewhere. Alternatively, the patient may seek no help.

Transference and Countertransference

Transference is the tendency we all have to see someone in the present as being like an important figure from our past. This process occurs outside our conscious awareness; it is probably a basic means used by the brain to make sense of current experience by seeing the past in the present and limiting the input of new information. Transference is more common in settings that provoke anxiety and provide few cues to how to behave – conditions typical of a hospital. Transference influences the patient's behavior and can distort the physician–patient relationship, for good or ill.

Although transference is a distortion of the present reality, it is usually built around a kernel of reality that can make it difficult for the inexperienced clinician to recognize rather than react to the transference. The transference can be the elaboration of an accurate observation into the "total" explanation or the major evidence of some expected harm or loss. Often the physician may recognize transference by the pressure she or he feels to respond in a particular manner to the patient, for example, always to stay longer or not abruptly leave the patient.

Transference is ubiquitous. It is a part of day-to-day experience, although its operation is outside conscious awareness. Recognizing transference in the physician–patient relationship can aid the physician in understanding the patient's deeply held expectations of help, shame, injury, or abandonment that derive from childhood experiences.

Transference reactions, of course, are not confined to the patient; the physician also superimposes the past on the present. This is called countertransference, the physician's transference to the patient (Table 2.2). Countertransference usually takes one of two forms: concordant countertransference, in which one empathizes with the patient's position; or complementary countertransference, in which one empathizes with an important figure from the patient's past. For example, concordant countertransference would be evident if a patient were describing an argument with his or her boss, and the psychiatrist, perhaps after a disagreement with the psychiatrist's own supervisor and without having collected detailed information from the patient, felt, "Oh yeah, what a terrible boss". Similarly, complementary countertransference would be evident if the same psychiatrist felt, "This person (the patient) does not work very hard, no wonder the boss is dissatisfied", and felt angry with the patient as well. Paying close attention to our personal reactions while refraining from immediate action can inform us in an experiential manner about subtle aspects of the patient's behavior that we may overlook or not appreciate. In the preceding example, the psychiatrist with the concordant countertransference might be identifying with the patient's subtle need to fight

Table 2.2 Types of Countertransference
Concordant countertransference
The physician experiences and empathizes with *the patient's* emotional experience and perception of reality
Complementary countertransference
The physician experiences and empathizes with the emotional experience and perception of reality of *an important person from the patient's life*

with authority. The psychiatrist with the complementary countertransference might have identified with the patient's boss, seeing only the patient's more passive wishes.

Countertransference occurs in all "sizes and shapes", more or less mixed with the physician's past but often greatly influencing the physician–patient relationship. The wish to save or rescue a patient is commonly experienced and indicates a need to look for countertransference responses. When a patient is seriously ill, such as with cancer, we may increasingly want to treat the patient more aggressively, with procedures that may hold little hope, create substantial pain, and perhaps even be against the patient's wishes. The physician's feelings of loss of a valued person (in the present and as a reminder of the past) or feelings of failure (loss of the physician's own power and ability) can often fuel such reactions. More subtle factors, such as the effects of being overworked, can result in unrecognized feelings of deprivation, leading to unspoken wishes for a patient to quit treatment. When these feelings appear in subtle countertransference reactions, such as being late to appointments, becoming tired in an hour, or being unable to recall previous material, they can have powerful effects on the patient's wish to continue treatment.

Major developmental events in physicians' lives can also influence their perceptions of their patients. When a psychiatrist is expecting the birth of a child, she or he may be overly sensitive to or ignore the concerns of a patient worried about a significant illness in the patient's child. Similarly, a physician with a dying parent or spouse may be unable to empathize with a patient's concerns about loss of a job, feeling that it is trivial (Clinical Vignette 5).

Clinical Vignette 5

A psychiatrist was called to evaluate an agitated older adult resident of a nursing home. After she had interviewed the energetic, sad, and anxious patient, the psychiatrist found herself unexpectedly sad, confused, and unsure about what to do. This was not a new case for the psychiatrist, who had treated many similar cases. In considering her response, her thoughts turned to her grandmother with whom she had lived when she was 8 years old, and who had been displaced from her residence and moved to a nursing home in another city by well-meaning children who wanted her near them. After the move, her grandmother had become depressed and disoriented and died 3 months later. The psychiatrist recalled feeling confused at the time of her grandmother's death, wondering why she had died when she had just moved to an attractive new home. Recalling her confusion, the psychiatrist could think more clearly about her present patient and wondered if the patient might be depressed. She talked further with the nurses and found symptoms of depression in addition to the nighttime agitation. This new information altered her decision on the type of medication to begin with and the need for psychotherapy in addition to medication.

Defense Mechanisms

All people, including patients, employ mechanisms of defense to protect themselves from the painful awareness of feelings and memories that can provoke overwhelming anxiety. Defense mechanisms are specific cognitive processes: ways of thinking that function in part to avoid painful feelings. They are often characteristic of a person and form a style of

Table 2.3 Common Defense Mechanisms

Healthier Defenses	More Primitive Defenses
Sublimation	Splitting
Humor	Projection
Repression	Projective identification
Displacement	Omnipotence
Intellectualization	Devaluing
Reaction formation	Primitive idealization
Reversal	Denial
Identification with the aggressor	Conversion
Asceticism	Avoidance
Altruism	
Isolation of affect	

cognition. Common defense mechanisms include projection, repression, displacement, intellectualization, humor, suppression, and altruism (Table 2.3).

Defense mechanisms may be more or less mature depending on the degree of distortion of reality and interpersonal disruption to which they lead. This patterning of feelings, thoughts, and behaviors by defense mechanisms is involuntary and arises in response to perceptions of anxiety or other emotional distress. The patient's characteristic defense mechanisms, the cognitive processes used to lower anxiety and unpleasant feelings, can greatly affect the physician–patient relationship. Defense mechanisms operate all the time; however, in times of high anxiety, such as in a hospital or during a life crisis, patients may become much less flexible in the defenses they use and may revert to using less mature defenses.

Clinical Vignettes 6 and 7 are examples of defense mechanisms (conversion and avoidance or repression) affecting the treatment relationship. In Clinical Vignette 6, the conversion reaction that resulted in the paralysis expressed both the patient's anger and his conflict over what to do. In Clinical Vignette 7, the physician knew that the forgetting was neither intentional nor conscious but was directed at denying the need for treatment. In these cases, recognizing the defenses was important to knowing how to relate to the patient (Clinical Vignette 6) and avoid a countertransference reaction of anger at the patient for lack of compliance (Clinical Vignette 7).

Mental Status of the Patient

The patient's mental status is a major determinant of the formation and nature of the relationship with the physician. A young, healthy patient with an acute disorder has different needs and expectations than a somewhat older person who comes for help with a condition that has been present for a number of years. Both differ from the older adult who comes to the physician expecting that the future will be filled with physical and emotional losses.

Clinical Vignette 6

A 36-year-old army first sergeant was hospitalized for the evaluation of acute paralysis of his right hand. When the results of a neurological workup revealed no evidence of organic pathology, psychiatric consultation was obtained. The patient denied any past psychiatric history or significant alcohol or other substance abuse. He described a healthy family support system but then hesitated, saying, "You know, Doc, there's one thing I just haven't been able to talk about with anyone". He proceeded to speak of the extreme pressure he was feeling on the job, where he had found out that his boss (the company commander) was behaving unethically. The patient stated, "I feel like I'm between a rock and a hard place – if I report it, I'm being disloyal to my boss, but if I don't, I'm betraying my soldiers and the army". After further elaborating his feelings of anger and disgust toward his boss, the patient asked to terminate the interview but agreed to talk with the psychiatrist again in the morning.

Returning the next morning, the psychiatrist was greeted by the patient, who was brushing his teeth, using his right hand. "Hey, Doc, I'm good to go!" The patient then described what happened the evening before. "I was telling my wife about how I've got to get out of here and get back to work, because, after all, I'm the commander's right-hand man. And you know what, Doc? My hand started to work! Get me out of here, I'm not crazy after all!" The patient then reviewed the process, aided by the psychiatrist, and was able to further his understanding of the link between his conflicted rage toward his boss and how it was expressed symbolically as an involuntary physical paralysis of his right hand. He resolved: "I'm gonna do the right thing. I got to live with myself", and planned to report the commander's misconduct on return to work. He was discharged from the hospital later that day, having regained full use of his hand.

Clinical Vignette 7

A 20-year-old man came for consultation because of uncertainty about his career. He soon revealed that he felt profoundly sad, hopeless, helpless, and even suicidal. He had a family history of depression. The physician and patient agreed to employ antidepressant medication aggressively. Yet, over a period of several weeks, the patient did not improve. When the physician asked why that might be happening, the patient revealed that he had frequently forgotten to take the prescribed medication and had forgotten to tell the physician that this was the case during two meetings. The physician explored the reasons for this, and together the physician and the patient learned that the patient felt ashamed of having been diagnosed as depressed and of having been considered to require medication. He felt he was not his own master and had experienced this as a severe blow to his self-esteem. Taking the medication was a reminder of this "flaw". Hearing himself say this and feeling the physician's empathic support, the patient recognized the irrationality of his behavior and felt relieved. In addition, the physician now understood better the intensity of the patient's feelings and changed the prescription to once-a-day dosage at bedtime to decrease the patient's sense of shame and increase compliance with the treatment.

It can be seen when comparing these two clinical vignettes (Clinical Vignettes 8 and 9) that the mental status of the patient helps define the nature of the physician–patient relationship, though in both cases the treatment relationship was of relatively brief duration and ended successfully.

Clinical Vignette 8

A 25-year-old recent law school graduate came to a psychiatrist following a romantic disappointment. He reported that he was very sad because his girlfriend had chosen to move to a different city, which he believed foretold the end of their relationship. He added that he had been having trouble sleeping for several weeks, and was worried because his exhaustion was causing problems in his ability to perform his work. When the physician took a careful history, he learned that this young man had led a successful life, and that his social and sexual development had been quite unremarkable. He had had good friends and close friendships, and several girlfriends in his life. He said he would miss his girlfriend, but that he never intended to marry her. The doctor indicated to her patient that sometimes, after such a disappointment, it was quite common for there to be a period of anxiety and that his sadness was a good sign, showing that he had a good capacity to attach and mourn the loss of a close friend. The psychiatrist also suggested that the patient may be more angry with the girlfriend than he had recognized, with which the patient agreed. The doctor prescribed a mild sleep medication, suggesting it may not even be required, and scheduled a follow-up appointment in a month. When the patient returned, he reported that he had used only two of the sleeping pills and had thrown the rest away. He did not want to schedule another appointment; he expressed gratitude to the psychiatrist and they parted company.

Clinical Vignette 9

A 70-year-old widowed lawyer was vigorous, active, and financially comfortable, with many friends and professional associates. She explained to the psychiatrist that the last year had, however, been very difficult for her. Six months before, her husband of 45 years had died after a 2-year struggle with congestive heart failure. She now found herself seriously depressed, despite her active life. She was thinking actively about giving up her law practice, though she was very involved in several ongoing cases, which she had previously found interesting and which held the promise of significant financial reward. She went on to say that she had no appetite. She was chronically sleep-deprived and was losing interest in her friends, children, and grandchildren. When taking a careful history, the psychiatrist also learned that this patient had suffered from a serious depression 35 years earlier, when she lost a pregnancy, and that this depression lasted for a year. It eventually resolved after she took a tricyclic antidepressant and engaged in brief, insight-oriented psychotherapy. In that therapy, her relationship with her own depressed mother had been discussed. With all this information, the psychiatrist suggested she and her patient meet weekly and that the treatment include a pharmacological intervention to help with the patient's current depression. This treatment ended successfully 1 year later.

The patient's mental status in this case was the focus of and major factor in the structure of a long psychotherapy that greatly assisted the rehabilitation of interpersonal skills and the understanding of his cognitive limitations and newly changed cognition. The ability to work with an empathic listener while confronting limitations and feelings of shame and embarrassment is a special opportunity of the well-formed doctor–patient relationship (Clinical Vignette 10).

Clinical Vignette 10

A 40-year-old man came to a psychiatrist with a long history of emotional difficulties. He had been a healthy and happy college student when he developed a skin abscess, which caused a septicemia and a brain infection. After this, his entire life changed. Although college was quite challenging, he was able to finish it, but had difficulty concentrating, his judgment was poor, and his impulse control impaired. He had difficulty remembering words, and he realized that his previously adequate social skills had been lost. Where once he had been charming and known for his sense of humor, he was now dull and in many ways boring. Yet there was more to him than that, and he longed for an opportunity to speak with an understanding listener in the hope that through such a relationship he might be able to make constructive changes in his life. He knew what had been lost, he wanted to understand his limitations better, and he wanted to be able to function well enough to keep a job. A more remote goal was to have a long-term relationship with a woman. His consulting psychiatrist knew that were she to take on this patient, it would be for the long haul. Fortunately, there were no financial barriers to treatment, and the pair worked together on a weekly basis for many years. In the course of that treatment, the patient came to understand the social situations that made him anxious and the way his emotional states of mind influenced changes in his cognitive function. He developed the ability to work and love more effectively; he met a woman who was kind and loving. The psychiatrist was invited to his wedding. She attended the religious service but quietly left the reception after congratulating her patient and his wife. By that time, years into the physician–patient relationship, the patient saw his physician as a wise observer, an advisor, and a trusted friend. To the physician, her patient was a happy reminder of how much a person can strive to improve his life, and a rich source of learning about the interaction of emotion, cognitive function, and behavior.

Special Issues in the Physician–Patient Relationship

Phase of Treatment

The treatment phase – early, middle, or late (Table 2.4) – affects the structure of the physician–patient relationship in terms of both the issues to be addressed and the task to be accomplished by the physician and the patient. The early stage of treatment involves developing a rapport, forming shared initial goals, and initiating the working alliance. Education of the patient is important to the success of the physician–patient relationship in this stage, so that the patient

Table 2.4	Key Features of Treatment Phases
Early: developing rapport, forming shared initial goals, initiating the working alliance	
Middle: refining shared goals, using a variety of trial interventions	
Late: assessing outcome, resolving presenting problems, planning for future	

Table 2.5	Factors Affecting the Physician–Patient Relationship
Phases of treatment: early, middle, late	
Treatment setting	
Transition between inpatient and outpatient treatment	
Managed care	
Health and illness of the physician	

learns what he or she can expect. In the middle stage of treatment, the physician and patient continuously refine their shared goals, and various interventions are tried. While this takes place, transference and countertransference are likely to emerge. How these are recognized and managed is critical to whether the relationship continues and is therapeutic.

In the later phase of treatment, the assessment of the outcome and plans for the future are the primary focus. The physician and the patient discuss the end of their relationship in a process known as termination. Successes and disappointments associated with the treatment are reviewed. The physician must be willing to acknowledge the patient's disappointments, as well as recognize her or his own disappointments in the treatment. The therapeutic alliance is strengthened in this stage when the physician accepts expressions of the patient's disappointments, encourages such expressions when they are not forthcoming, and prepares the patient for the future. Such preparations include orienting the patient as to when he or she might seek further treatment. Solidifying the physician–patient relationship at the end of the treatment can be critical to the patient's self-esteem and willingness to return if symptoms reappear (Table 2.5).

As a part of the termination process, the physician and the patient must review what has been learned, discuss what changes have taken place in the patient and the patient's life, and acknowledge together the sadness and joy of their leave-taking. The termination involves a mourning process even when treatment has been brief or unpleasant. Of course, when the physician–patient relationship has been rewarding, and both physician and patient are satisfied with what they have accomplished, mourning is more intense and often characterized by a bittersweet sadness.

Treatment Settings

The physician–patient relationship takes place in a variety of treatment settings. These include the private office, community clinic, emergency room, inpatient psychiatric ward, and general hospital ward. Psychiatrists treating patients in a private office may find that the relative privacy of this setting enhances the early establishment of trust related to confidentiality. In addition, the psychiatrist's personality is more evident in the private office where personal factors influencing choice of decor, room arrangement, and location play a role. However, in contrast to the hospital or community setting, the private office generally lacks other evidence of the physician's competence and humanness. In hospital and community settings, when a colleague greets the physician and the patient in the hall, or the physician receives a call for a consultation by a colleague or for a meeting, it indicates to the patient that the physician is qualified, skilled, and humane.

On the other hand, therapeutic work conducted in the community clinic, emergency room, and general hospital ward often requires the psychiatrist and patient to adapt rapidly to meeting one another, assessing the problem, establishing treatment goals, and ensuring the appropriate interventions and follow-up. The importance of protecting the patient's needs for time, predictability, and structure can run counter to the demands of a busy service and unexpected clinical and administrative requirements. The psychiatrist must stay alert to the patient's perspective but not all interruptions can be avoided. The patient can be informed and accommodated as much as possible, and any feelings of hurt, disappointment, or anger can be listened for by the physician and responded to empathically. At times, patients, particularly those with borderline personality disorder, may require transfer to another psychiatrist whose schedule can accommodate the patient's exquisite needs for stability.

The boundaries of confidentiality are necessarily extended in hospital and community settings to include consultation with other physicians, nursing staff, and often family members. Particular attention must always be given to the patient's need for and right to respect and privacy. Regardless of the setting, patients receiving medication must be fully informed about the potential risks and benefits of and alternatives to the recommended pharmacological treatment. Patients must be educated about the risks and benefits of receiving prescribed treatment and of not receiving treatment. This is an important component of maintaining the physician–patient relationship. Patients who are informed about and involved in decisions about medication respect the physician's role and interest in their welfare. Psychiatrists must also pay particular attention to the meaning a patient attaches to any prescribed medication, particularly when the time comes to alter or discontinue its use.

The change from inpatient to outpatient therapy involves the resumption of a greater degree of autonomy by the patient in the physician–patient dyad. The physician must actively encourage this separation and its hope for the future. This transition is delicate for any therapeutic pair.

The Physician–Patient Relationship in Specific Populations of Patients

Cross-cultural and Ethnic Issues

Addressing cross-cultural issues such as race, ethnicity, religion, and gender is vital to the establishment and maintenance of an effective physician–patient relationship (see Chapter 3). Failure to clarify cultural assumptions, whether stemming from differences or similarities in background, may impede the establishment of a trusting therapeutic alliance, making effective treatment unlikely.

Children, Adolescents, and Families

Establishing an effective physician–patient relationship with children, adolescents, and families is one of the most challenging and rewarding tasks in the practice of psychiatry. Rather than being treated as "little adults", children and adolescents must be approached with an appreciation for their age-appropriate developmental tasks and needs. When physicians treat this population, they must establish a trusting relationship with both the patient and the parents. Preadolescent children face the psychosocial developmental tasks of establishing trust, autonomy, initiative, and achievement. By understanding the facets of normal childhood development, physicians may help parents understand the nature of their child's disturbance and work within the family system to establish effective mechanisms for coping and recovery.

Adolescent patients, facing the task of establishing an individual identity, pose particular challenges to the physician–patient relationship. Adolescents are particularly sensitive to any signals from the physician that their powers of decision, their intelligence, or their perceptions are being ignored. Defiance, detachment, and aggression may be anticipated and defused with a steady therapeutic presence grounded in consistent boundaries and open acknowledgment of the adolescent patient's distress.

In working with families, physicians in general and psychiatrists in particular must clearly address questions and concerns regarding all aspects of treatment and convey respectful compassion for all members. The therapeutic alliance, or "joining" with the family and patient, requires developing enough of a family consensus that treatment is worth the struggle involved. Taking sides and engaging with individual and family power struggles can be particularly destructive to the physician–patient relationship in families.

Terminally Ill Patients

Terminally ill patients share concerns related to the end of the life cycle. Elderly patients at all levels of health face the developmental task of integrating the various threads of their life into a figurative tapestry that reflects their lifelong feelings, thoughts, values, goals, beliefs, experiences, and relationships, and places them into a meaningful perspective. Patients newly diagnosed with a terminal illness such as metastatic cancer or acquired immunodeficiency syndrome may be particularly overwhelmed and initially unable to deal with the demands of their illness, especially if the patient is a young adult or child. Psychiatrists may enhance the terminally ill patient's ability to cope by addressing issues related to medical treatment, pharmacotherapy, psychotherapy, involvement of significant others, legal matters, and institutional care. Patients struggling with spiritual or religious concerns may benefit from a religious consultation, a resource that is frequently unused.

Countertransference feelings ranging from fear to helplessness to rage to despair can assist the therapist greatly in maintaining the physician–patient relationship and ensuring appropriate care. Issues commonly encountered with disabled patients include inaccurate assumptions about their ability to function fully in all areas of human activity, including sex and vocation. Terminally ill patients may evoke reactions of unwarranted pessimism, thwarting the physician's ability to help the patient maximize hope for the quality of whatever time may remain. Patients and their family members often look to their physician for guidance.

Conclusion

The physician–patient relationship is essential to the healing process and is the foundation on which an effective treatment plan may be negotiated, integrating the best of what medical technology and human caring can provide. The centrality of this relationship is particularly true for psychiatric physicians and their patients. In the psychiatrist–patient relationship, empathy, compassion, and hope frequently serve as the major means of alleviating pain and enhancing active participation in all treatment interventions: biological, psychological, and social.

The development of the physician–patient relationship depends on skilled assessment, the development of rapport through empathy, a strong therapeutic alliance, and the effective understanding of transference, countertransference, and defense mechanisms. Current research findings support the purposeful use of common therapy factors, of which the therapeutic alliance is the most powerful, to enhance clinical outcome.

The development of the physician–patient relationship is influenced by numerous factors, including the phase of treatment, the treatment setting, transitions between inpatient and outpatient care, managed care, and changes in the physician's health. The astute physician is attuned to the needs and characteristics of specific populations of patients, adopting the therapeutic approach that most effectively bridges the gap between physician and patient and leads to a healing relationship.

References

Petrovic P, Kalso E, Petersson KM *et al.* (2002) Placebo and opioid analgesia – Imaging a shared neuronal network. *Science* 295, 1737–1740.

Ursano RJ and Silberman EK (1988) Individual psychotherapies, in *The American Psychiatric Press Textbook of Psychiatry* (eds Talbott JA, Hales RE and Yudofsky SC). American Psychiatric Press, Washington, DC, pp. 876–884.

CHAPTER

3 The Cultural Context of Clinical Assessment

Introduction: The Cultural Matrix of Psychiatry

Although it has long been recognized that the mode of expressing psychological distress and behavioral disturbances varies with cultural beliefs and practices, a growing body of evidence shows that the effects of culture are more far-reaching. It is well established that the causes, course, and outcome of major psychiatric disorders are influenced by cultural factors. Wide variations in the prevalence of many psychiatric disorders across geographic regions and ethnocultural groups have been documented with current standardized epidemiological survey methods. In addition, social and cultural factors are major determinants of the use of health-care services and alternative sources of help.

For all of these reasons, careful assessment of the cultural context of psychiatric problems must form a central part of any clinical evaluation. Beyond this, culturally based attitudes and assumptions govern the perspectives that both patient and clinician bring to the clinical encounter. Lack of awareness of important differences can undermine the development of a therapeutic alliance and the negotiation and delivery of effective treatment.

The changing demography of North America and around the world has made the recognition and response to cultural diversity increasingly important in psychiatric practice. Sociological research has shown a high degree of retention of ethnic culture with the persistence of religious practices, family life-cycle rituals, and ethnic enclaves in many cities. Added to this is the recognition of the importance of maintaining and renewing ethnocultural identity to combat the legacy of racial discrimination. This has led to rethinking the notion of assimilation to take into account other modes of acculturation including the development of multiple cultural identities. More recent waves of global migration from south to north and east to west have brought together new mixes of peoples with greater differences in their cultural assumptions, with corresponding challenges for intercultural clinical work.

These changes, along with larger forces of globalization, have encouraged a fresh look at culture in every area of psychiatry. In clinical practice, "cultural competence" has become the

The Psychiatric Interview: Evaluation and Diagnosis, First Edition. Allan Tasman, Jerald Kay and Robert J. Ursano.

This chapter is based on Chapter 4 (Laurence J. Kirmayer, Cécile Rousseau, G. Eric Jarvis, Jaswant Guzder) of *Psychiatry*, 3rd Edition.

rubric under which to advance a broad range of skills and perspectives pertinent to working with a culturally diverse clinical population. In the sections that follow, we will summarize some of the concepts and approaches that can inform culturally competent clinical practice.

What Is Culture?

There is a famous saying to the effect that we do not know who discovered water but it was not the fish. So it is with culture: we are immersed in our own cultural worlds from birth, and consequently our culture is largely implicit and unexamined. Just as we are unconscious of many of our own motivations and patterns of thought and behavior until they are reflected back to us by others, so too are we unconscious of our cultural background knowledge and assumptions. Bringing the cultural unconscious to light may be more difficult than facing the individual unconscious because institutions and others around us may reinforce our assumptions and resist any attempt to question them. Our explicit appreciation of culture usually comes from intercultural encounters, which make us suddenly aware of culture through difference. More formally, anthropological research comparing different cultures allows us to see the tacit assumptions of our own worldviews. Older views of culture were based on ethnographic studies of relatively isolated small-scale societies. Many accounts tended to assume that cultures were finely balanced systems and that, as a result, everything was for a purpose and had an adaptive function for the group (if not always for the individual). The outsider was thus cautioned not to pass judgment on cultural differences or to see pathology where there was simply difference. This is still wise advice. However, it is clear that cultures are not homeostatic systems in a steady state or equilibrium but are constantly shifting and evolving systems. They may be riven by conflict and create maladaptive circumstances not only for disadvantaged individuals but for specific groups or even the society as a whole. Thus, while refraining from prejudging specific cultural values or practices, the clinician must nevertheless consider that every culture encompasses practices that may help or hinder patients, and aggravate or ameliorate any given type of psychopathology. Each society tends to cultivate blind spots around the specific forms of social suffering that it produces (Kleinman *et al.*, 1997). Openness, respect, and capacity for collective self-criticism are thus key elements of any transcultural clinical encounter.

At the same time, anthropologists have come to recognize the high level of individual variability within even small cultural groups and the active ways in which individuals and groups make use of a variety of forms of knowledge to fashion an identity and a viable way of living. In urban settings where many cultures meet, individuals have a wide range of options available and can position themselves both within and against any given ethnocultural identity or way of living. This has led anthropologists to rethink the notion of culture or even to suggest that it has outlived its usefulness.

Indeed, the modern world includes forms of electronic communication and rapid transportation that have begun to weave the whole globe together in new ways. This results in the intermixing of cultural worlds and the creation of new ethnocultural groups and individuals with multiple or hybrid identities. Many people now see themselves as transnational, with networks of affiliation and support that span great distances. The mental health implications of these new forms of identity and community have been inadequately explored and will be an increasingly important issue for psychiatry.

As this brief discussion makes clear, the notion of culture covers a broad territory. It is useful precisely because of this breadth, but to apply it to clinical practice, we need to make some further specifications and distinctions. In the North American context, it is useful to distinguish notions of race, ethnicity, and social class from culture.

Race is a term used to mark off groups within and between societies. Racial distinctions generally reflect a few superficial physical characteristics and hence have little correlation with clinically relevant genetic variation. Race is usually ascribed by others and cannot readily be changed or discarded unless larger social criteria change. Race is significant as a social category that is employed in racist and discriminatory practices. Racism is clinically important because of its effects on mental and physical health and the challenge it presents to both individual and collective self-esteem.

Ethnicity refers to the collective identity of a group based on common heritage, which may include language, religion, geographic origin, and specific cultural practices. Ethnic identity is often constructed vis-à-vis others and a dominant society. Hence, it is sometimes assumed that "foreigners" or minorities have ethnicity while the dominant group (e.g., Americans of British or northern European extraction) does not. This obscures the fact that everyone may become aware of an ethnic identity in the right context (in China, an American clearly has a distinct ethnicity). Ethnicity may be chosen or ascribed by others. For example, the US census defined five ethnoracial blocs: White, African-American, Hispanic, Asian-American and Pacific Islander, and American Indian and Alaska Native. These are heterogeneous categories variously based on race, language, geographic origin, and ethnicity, but they have acquired practical and political reality because they have been used to present epidemiological findings and define health service needs. Nevertheless, the clinician must recognize that to meet the patient on a common ground requires a much more fine-grained notion of ethnocultural identity than afforded by these crude categories.

Finally, social class reflects the fact that most societies are economically stratified and individuals' opportunities, mobility, lifestyle, and response to illness are heavily constrained by their economic position. Issues of poverty, unemployment, powerlessness, and marginalization may overshadow cultural factors as causes of illness and influences on identity and help-seeking behavior. Violence is a particularly striking example in North American society of the overlap of exclusion, poverty, discrimination, and intergenerational transmission of trauma.

The notion of culture is sometimes extended to speak of various subcultures or the cultures of professions. In this sense, we can speak of the cultures of biomedicine and of psychiatry. Each of these systems of knowledge includes a wide range of behavioral norms and institutional practices that may be familiar to clinicians but novel and confusing to patients. However, familiar cultural notions of self and personhood underwrite these technical domains, and therefore serve to reinforce larger cultural ideologies. This becomes clear when we consider alternative systems of medicine such as traditional Chinese medicine or Indian Ayurveda, which are based on different notions of the person (ethnopsychology), the body (ethnophysiology), and different roles for patient and healer. Even the understanding and practice of biomedicine may differ across countries, so the clinician should not assume that familiar terms always refer to the same practice.

Culture and Gender

Gender refers to the ways in which cultures differentiate and define roles based on biological sex or reproductive functions. Because of this link with physical aspects of sex, there is a tendency to view gender differences as biological givens, though cultural beliefs also play a role.

Men and women do have some fundamentally different experiences of their bodies, of their social worlds, and of their life course. It has been suggested that women are more in touch with their bodies because of the experiences of menstruation, childbearing, childbirth, breast-feeding, and menopause. These differences may be as substantial as any between disparate cultures. At the same time, there is much evidence that these bodily grounded experiences vary substantially across cultures. There are also important gender differences in styles of emotional expression, symptom experience, and help-seeking. In epidemiological surveys in the USA, women tend to report more somatic symptoms as well as more emotional distress, and they are more likely to seek help for psychological or interpersonal problems. However, the gender difference in symptom reporting varies significantly cross-nationally.

In North America, important differences have been documented in male and female styles of conversation that are relevant to the clinical context. In general, women tend to give more frequent acknowledgments that they are listening to a speaker. They may give signs of assent simply to indicate they are following the conversation. Men tend to be more taciturn and, if they signal assent, it usually means they actually agree with the speaker. These differences in communication style may lead to systematic misunderstandings between men and women that are further aggravated by cultural differences in gender roles and etiquette (Clinical Vignette 1).

Clinical Vignette 1

When an ultra-orthodox Jewish family arrives for their consultation, the female psychiatrist, who is dressed in a short skirt, welcomes them offering her hand to the father in greeting. He is confused and offended, avoiding eye contact and reluctant to proceed with the session. The female doctor's style of dress and friendly handshake were viewed as disrespectful or as indicating her lack of familiarity with norms of conduct with observant orthodox families.

In many societies, gender is associated with marked differences in power and social status. For example, in patriarchal societies, men have specific power and privileges that give them a measure of control over the lives of women. This is often coupled with responsibilities for maintaining family honor and well-being. In recent years, North American society has espoused social and political equality in gender roles. From this egalitarian point of view, patriarchal families may seem oppressive to women. However, women may accept and participate in cultural definitions of their roles that appear restrictive by North American cultural norms but that make family life meaningful. Any judgment as to whether a given family's relationships are oppressive or pathological must not only take into account social norms and practices but also explore the meaning of issues and events for the individuals involved (Clinical Vignette 2).

Clinical Vignette 2

A 29-year-old East Indian woman, in the USA for 6 months, presents with symptoms of depression and posttraumatic stress disorder (PTSD). Throughout the initial evaluation, the patient looks away from the male psychiatrist, never making eye contact. The interviewer is concerned that he may have offended the woman in some way. The female interpreter explains that the patient is showing respect by not looking directly at a male in authority.

Differences in cultural definitions of gender roles may become sources of conflict after migration. Culturally prescribed patterns of marriage and childbearing may be central to the social status, identity, and self-esteem of men and women even when they are not given the same importance in the dominant culture (Clinical Vignette 3).

Clinical Vignette 3

A 28-year-old woman from South Asia has an arranged marriage with an older man from the same religious community, who has lived all of his life in the USA. The couple has been unable to conceive for 5 years and is in the midst of extensive infertility treatments. The husband complains that she is paranoid and does not want to work or go out of the house. The woman tearfully relates that she feels depressed and ashamed because of her predicament and fears that her marriage will end if she cannot bear children.

The Cultural Formulation

In an effort to address the cultural dimensions of clinical assessment, DSM-IV-TR introduced an outline for a cultural formulation. This outline covers major areas that a clinician should explore in a comprehensive evaluation for every patient and includes gaining an understanding of the individual's identity and explanation for the illness, their environment, and social situation, and other typical aspects of a thorough evaluation such as the way the patient interacts with the clinician (American Psychiatric Association, 1994). The complete formulation may go well beyond the DSM-IV-TR categories to consider many sorts of problems and predicaments relevant to the patient's well-being.

The cultural formulation is merely intended as a checklist or reminder to encourage the clinician to perform the needed exploration and integration of a broad range of relevant social and cultural information. Clearly, cultural considerations may apply to every aspect of the clinical assessment and interview and must not be used only as an afterthought to the standard psychiatric interview.

Ethnocultural Identity

The first dimension of the cultural formulation involves ethnocultural identity. This includes the individual's ethnic or cultural reference groups and the position of these groups vis-à-vis the larger society. Certain groups have a specific ethnocultural identity ascribed to them by others; this may have an impact on individuals' everyday experience and narratives of identity, whether or not they are explicitly aware of it.

In a world of mass migration and intermingling of peoples over generations, identity is very often hybrid, and not specifically determined by one's ethnic or cultural heritage. For immigrant and ethnic minorities, it is important to understand the degree of involvement with both the culture of origin and the host culture. Ethnic identity may be situational and shift with social context. The ethnocultural and religious groups with which the patient most identifies may depend on who asks the question and in what context. For example, whether someone self-identifies as Canadian, West Indian, or Trinidadian may depend on the perceived identity of the interviewer and the setting where the interview takes place.

Language is central to identity for many people and has a profound effect on clinical encounters. Individuals who speak multiple languages, learned at different stages in their life, may have different memories, affects, and interpersonal schemas associated with the use of each language. Languages may be associated with developmentally important relationships and tied to specific areas of conflict or mastery. Personal and political allegiances within the family and community may be expressed through choice of language.

Language is the medium through which experience is articulated; hence, the assessment of higher cognitive functions, complex emotions, and experiential symptoms of pathology all depend on the clinician's access to the patient's language. Patients who are hobbled in a second language may be misjudged as less intelligent or competent than they are in fact; wishing to avoid such bias, clinicians may be overly generous in their assessment and miss significant problems or pathology.

Even where patients have a moderate level of facility in the clinician's preferred language, they may not express themselves fully in a second language so that important details are not conveyed. The use of a second language not only affects doctor–patient communication, it also influences individuals' ability to reflect about themselves. When patients are forced to formulate their problems in a language in which they are not proficient, they may be less creative and effective as problem solvers. When patients are able to use their own best language, their accounts of experience become much richer, more complex, and nuanced; their thinking is subtler; they can express a wider range of affect and engage in playful therapeutic exchanges.

Multilingual people sometimes report that they feel and think differently when using a second language. In part, this is due to the cognitive effort of having to find words in a language in which one is not totally fluent. Since each language favors certain modes of expression and ways of thinking, bilingual speakers may report that they feel like a different person in their other language. It follows that aspects of the history and experience of a patient can be less accessible in a clinical evaluation if patients are not able to express themselves in the appropriate language. Of course, use of a second language may also afford the patient some distance from intense emotions and painful memories, and so assist in coping and affect regulation. Careful attention to spontaneous or strategic shifts in use of language in a multilingual assessment can provide the clinician with important information about areas of conflict and strengths. Often this requires the use of a trained interpreter, as discussed later in this chapter.

Religion is another key marker of identity. For many individuals and communities, it may structure the moral world more strongly than ethnic or national identity. The term "spirituality" has gained currency to acknowledge the fact that many individuals maintain deeply held personal beliefs about God, the meaning of life, and what happens after death, without being formally affiliated with one religion or another. Religious affiliation is also a frequent source of discrimination.

Despite the ubiquity of religious and spiritual experience, it is frequently neglected during routine psychiatric evaluation. A thorough cultural formulation requires consideration of the patient's religion and spirituality. Areas to cover include religious identity, the role of religion in the family of origin, current religious practices (attendance at services, public and private rituals), motivation for religious behavior (i.e., religious orientation), and specific beliefs of individuals and of their family and community.

Illness Explanations and Help-Seeking

The second major dimension of the cultural formulation concerns cultural explanations of symptoms and illness. Cultures provide systems of diagnosis and treatment of illness and affliction that may influence patients' experience of illness and help-seeking behavior. People label and interpret their distress based on these systems of knowledge, which they share with others around them. Much research in medical anthropology has developed the idea of explanatory models, which may include accounts of causality, mechanism or process, course, appropriate treatment, expected outcome, and consequences. Not all of this knowledge is related directly to personal experience – much of it resides in cultural knowledge and practices carried out by others. Hence, understanding the cultural meanings of symptoms and behavior may require interviews with other people in the patient's family, entourage, or community.

It is also important to ask questions for eliciting patients' explanatory models. These questions should be modified based on the patient's responses. For example, the origins of problems may be located not in the body but in the workings of the mind, the family, the community, the realms of ancestors or spirits, or in mythological accounts that explain the social and moral order. For example, a patient may feel that someone has used a religious procedure to place a curse on them.

In many cases, particularly with acute illness, patients may not have well-developed explanatory models. Instead, they reason by analogy on the basis of past experiences of their own or other prominent prototypes encountered in family, friends, or mass media. Once an explanatory model is evoked in conversation, however, patients may give formulaic accounts that accord with that cultural model or script. Therefore, to obtain more complete information about the cognitive and social factors that are actually influencing the patients' illness experience and behavior, it is useful to begin with an open-ended interview that simply aims to reconstruct the events surrounding symptoms and the illness experience. This will reveal idiosyncratic temporal patterns of contiguity and association that may not fit any explicit cultural model. Following this, the clinician can ask about prototypes (Have you ever had anything like this before? Has anyone you know ever had anything like this before?). This will uncover salient models of illness that may shape illness experience and be used to reason analogically about the current episode. Finally, it is important to inquire into explicit cultural models using the sorts of questions devised for the explanatory model interview.

The ethnomedical systems described in anthropological texts often are idealized and complex portraits pieced together by working with cultural experts. In clinical practice, patients usually have only partial or fragmentary knowledge of the traditional explanations and treatment for their problem. Depending on the knowledge and attitudes of family and kin, and on the availability of practitioners of traditional medical systems, patients may be influenced by larger cultural systems to which they themselves do not fully subscribe.

In everyday life, people use culturally prescribed idioms to discuss their problems. These cultural idioms of distress cut across specific diagnostic categories. They may be used to talk about ordinary problems as well as to shape the expression of distress associated with major psychiatric disorders. For example, many cultures have notions of "nerves" (in Spanish, *nervios*), which signal emotional distress that may range from mild upset with life events to disabling anxiety or psychosis. Appendix I of DSM-IV-TR provides a list of some common idioms of distress. The same appendix also lists some well-described culture-bound syndromes, culturally distinctive clusters of symptoms that may be of pathological significance. Many culture-specific terms, however, do not refer to syndromes or idioms of distress but are actually symptoms or illness attributions that reference folk models of causality. For example, *susto*, a term used in Central and South America, attributes a wide range of bodily symptoms and diseases (including infectious diseases and congenital malformations) to the damaging effects of sudden fright (Clinical Vignette 4).

Clinical Vignette 4

A family from Nigeria consults for developmental delay in their 4-year-old son. Problems had become evident when they attempted to integrate the child into a preschool program. The child presents a classical profile of pervasive developmental disorder. The parents comment that their family doctor raised the possibility of autism but that they did not consider that what he described applied to their son. They explain that the migration process, when the child was 2, had hindered his acquisition of speech and social activities. After a few sessions, it becomes apparent that the child's difficulties had already been recognized in Nigeria but were attributed by both the maternal and the paternal lineage to sorcery on the other side of the family because they were in conflict.

Many cultural idioms of distress use bodily metaphors for experience. In seeking medical help, patients usually try to present the sort of problems they believe the clinician is competent to treat. Consequently, in biomedical settings, patients tend to emphasize physical symptoms. The social stigma commonly associated with psychiatric symptoms and disorders, as well as with substance abuse, antisocial behavior, and various other behaviors also may prevent patients from acknowledging such problems and events. However, with clear communication and a respectful stance, the clinician may be able to build sufficient trust over time for patients to disclose shameful or potentially stigmatizing information.

Similarly, people commonly use multiple remedies or consult various healers for their symptoms, and may be reluctant to disclose treatments they think the clinician will not understand or accept. They may also omit mention of preparations they view as "natural" or as foods and hence not included under the rubric of medications or drugs. A nonjudgmental inquiry by the clinician will enable patients to discuss more freely their use of traditional and alternative treatments.

Psychosocial Environment and Levels of Functioning

Cultural factors have a dual influence on the psychosocial environment: they determine life circumstances and, at the same time, provide interpretations of their meaning and significance for the individual. This dual effect of culture means that the clinician must explore both events and their personal and cultural meanings to understand the impact of the social environment.

There are wide cultural variations in the composition and functioning of families, including the variety of people living together in a household (not always identical to the family or kin); who is considered close or distant kin; hierarchy, power structure, and economic arrangements; age and gender roles; organization of household activities and routines; styles of expression of emotion and distress; body practices (arrangements and procedures for sleeping, eating, washing, dressing, recreation, and use of physical remedies for ailments); conflict management strategies; and the relationship of family to larger social networks and communities.

Social support must be assessed with attention to cultural configurations of the family and community. Extended multigenerational families, tightly knit religious and ethnocultural communities, and transnational networks all may provide specific forms of instrumental and emotional support. Often these supports are inextricably intertwined with interpersonal obligations and demands that may constitute burdens for the individual. This complex relationship of burden and support may have crucial implications for clinical interventions (Clinical Vignette 5).

Clinical Vignette 5

A woman from South Asia appears to have a severe depression with vegetative symptoms and persistent suicidal ideation. She does not respond to trials of several antidepressant medications. On reassessment with a clinician who speaks her language, she reveals that her husband has an unpaid debt of honor to her daughter's husband's family, and she is suffering from the ongoing feud, which has barred her from seeing her daughter and grandchildren. When this is addressed in a series of family therapy sessions, her "depression" lifts dramatically.

Similarly, levels of functioning and disability must be assessed against culturally determined notions of social roles and values. It is important to recognize that the clinician's priority may not be the most important issue for patients or their families.

In addition to these general cultural considerations, certain social situations present specific stressors with which the clinician must become familiar. All immigrants and refugees arrive in the host country after a migration experience. For some, migration is a personal choice taken in the hope of bettering personal and family prospects; for others, the experience is borne of extreme difficulty and is only taken under threat of harm or death. Many new arrivals face bleak job prospects, are isolated from family and cultural institutions, and have an uphill battle as they adapt to a new language and unfamiliar social rules and obligations. Furthermore, the path that some immigrants take prior to arriving at their final destination is often lengthy, circuitous, and costly, in addition to being dangerous. It is crucial, therefore, to take into account the migration experience when evaluating immigrants and refugees. Questions must be carefully phrased and asked in a judicious manner, as not all patients will be ready to discuss their reasons for leaving their homeland. Important points to cover include the premigration lifestyle of the patient, the context of migration, the experience of migration, the postmigration experience, and the "aftermath" of migration, or the long-term adjustment and acculturation to the host society.

The stresses experienced by refugees may include the confusion and disorientation of unplanned flight and exile; loss of social status, wealth, security, and community; and worry about the safety of family left behind and still in peril. Refugee claimants or asylum seekers usually face a stressful period of uncertainty while waiting to have their status determined (Clinical Vignette 6).

Clinical Vignette 6

A 35-year-old professional from Peru visited the emergency room because of high fever caused by pneumonia. While waiting to be seen, he suddenly became agitated and fled the hospital, breaking through the parking lot barrier. After his arrest the judge ordered a psychiatric assessment. The patient explained that on seeing the medical instruments in the ER, he was reminded of his torture in Peru and felt convinced that he was back there and that his life was in danger. The combined effects of fever and reminders of the trauma had triggered a dissociative episode.

In addition, the growing number of undocumented people around the world also presents ethical and pragmatic challenges to the medical profession. These illegal immigrants and families may have particular mental health needs, which are largely unrecognized because there is almost no funded research or services to address them.

Clinician–Patient Relationship

The roles of healer, helper, and physician differ across cultural contexts, and patients may have correspondingly different expectations of their relationship with clinicians, including the duration, level of disclosure, formality, and emphasis on technical competence. These expectations often need to be explored, with opportunities for patients and clinicians to negotiate or explain limits to the roles they are able and willing to adopt. Once these differing perspectives are made explicit, a culturally appropriate and professionally acceptable relationship and working alliance can be negotiated. Clinicians must become aware of their own ethnocultural background and identity and reflect on how it is perceived by patients from their own and different backgrounds (Clinical Vignette 7).

Clinical Vignette 7

On the recommendation of her 8-year-old son's school, a university-educated woman from Somalia consults for his conduct problems, which are not responding to stimulant medication prescribed by a pediatrician for attention deficit hyperactivity disorder. She is obviously reticent about the assessment process. The white clinician explicitly addresses the difficulty of being a black, veiled woman in North America because of the strong prejudices against both Islam and Africa. The woman visibly relaxes and begins to explain that she feels that she is being treated as though she is intellectually handicapped or as a child by the school. They use a loud voice and simplistic formulations when they speak to her, and she finds this very humiliating. Later in the interview, after further strengthening of the alliance with the clinician, she discloses the war trauma to which the boy was exposed.

Overall Assessment

The aim of the cultural assessment is to integrate all of the pertinent elements of the cultural context of the patient's identity, illness, and social context in a formulation that can guide diagnosis and treatment. Factors associated with one aspect of the formulation may have an impact that cuts across many dimensions of illness experience and behavior. The salient aspects of culture vary across cases and may reflect issues in the dominant society as much as any intrinsic characteristics of the patient's ethnocultural group.

For example, cultural notions of race and racism may profoundly affect every aspect of the cultural formulation.

Cultural Competence

Recent years have seen the development of professional standards for training and quality assurance in cultural competence. This term stands for a range of approaches aimed at improving the delivery of appropriate services to a culturally diverse population. This includes the clinician's ability to elicit cultural information during the clinical encounter (Table 3.1), to understand how different cultural worlds of patients and their families influence the course of the illness, and to develop a treatment plan that empowers the patient by acknowledging cultural knowledge and resources while allowing appropriate psychiatric intervention.

Table 3.1 Strategies to Elicit Cultural Information
• Present an open, friendly face of the institution (have the diversity of the community represented within the diversity of the institution, with attention to not simply reproducing the class structure of the society in the institutional hierarchy). • Make explicit the clinician's position and identity, explain goals and methods, use self-disclosure appropriately. • Ask for clarification of unfamiliar terms or key terms that may be mistakenly assumed to be familiar. • Ask for detailed description of practices related to health, illness, and coping. • Have the patient compare situation with previous events or experiences of others from similar background. • Interview other family members and patient's entourage to obtain normative framework and identify consensus and conflicting perspectives. • Consult knowledgeable clinicians, culture-brokers, interpreters, anthropologists, and ethnographic literature.

Specific cultural competence has to do with knowledge and skills pertaining to a single cultural group, which may include history, language, etiquette, styles of child-rearing, emotional expression, and interpersonal interaction as well as cultural explanations of illness and specific modalities of healing. Often, it is assumed that specific cultural competence is assured when there is an ethnic match between clinician and patient (e.g., a Hispanic clinician treating a client from the same background). However, ethnic matching without explicit training in models of culture and intercultural interaction may not be sufficient to ensure that clinicians become aware of their tacit cultural knowledge or biases and apply their cultural skills in a clinically effective manner (Clinical Vignette 8).

Clinical Vignette 8

A 16-year-old girl from Haiti presents with disorganized schizophrenia, which began around age 14 years. Her family has not been compliant with treatment and this had led to several hospitalizations of the patient in a dehydrated state. During the third hospitalization, the clinical team decides to explore the family's interpretation of the illness. A grand-aunt insists on sending the girl to Haiti for a traditional diagnosis. The traditional healer indicates that the problem is due to an ancestor's spirit in the mother's family and that for this reason it will be a prolonged illness. This explanation helps to restore cohesion in the extended family by rallying people around the patient, and her family receives much support. The traditional interpretation and treatment have broken the family sense of shame and isolation and promoted an alliance with the medical team and the acceptance of antipsychotic medication.

At the level of the individual, it may be easier to establish rapport when clinician and patient share a common background. However, there is a risk that some issues may be left unexplored because they are taken for granted, or are taboo and awkward to approach. There is also difficulty when the patient's expectations of a fellow community member are not met because the clinician applies the rules and limits dictated by professional training. This may include expectations of receiving special treatment, of being cured quickly, of becoming friends, or intervening inappropriately on behalf of other family or community members.

In many cases, however, ethnic matching is only crude or approximate. For example, the term "Hispanic" covers a broad territory with many cultural, educational, and social class differences that transcend language. Indeed, there is enormous intracultural variation and no one person carries comprehensive knowledge of his or her own cultural background, so there is always the need to explore local meanings with patients.

In the course of professional training, clinicians may distance themselves from their own culture of origin and become reluctant or unable to use (or understand the impact of) their tacit cultural knowledge in their clinical work. Clinicians from ethnic minority backgrounds may resent being pigeon-holed and expected to work predominately with a specific ethnocultural group. Patients may have complex reactions to meeting a clinician from the same background. These issues require attention and sensitive exploration just as much as the feelings evoked by meeting someone from a different background.

At the level of technique, the clinician familiar with a specific ethnocultural group learns to modify his or her approach to take advantage of culturally supported coping strategies. For example, religious practices, family and community supports, and appeals to specific cultural values may all provide useful strategies for symptom management and improved functioning. Traditional diagnostic and treatment methods may be used in concert with conventional psychiatric treatments. The clinician may use his or her own person differently in recognition of cultural notions of healing relationships, adopting a more authoritative stance, making selective use of self-disclosure, or participating in symbolic social exchanges with patients and their extended families to establish trust and credibility.

Increasingly, clinicians work in settings where there is great cultural diversity that precludes reaching a high level of specific competence for any one group. Changes in migration patterns and new waves of immigrants and refugees lead to corresponding changes in patient populations. For all of these reasons, it is crucial to supplement specific cultural competence with more generic competence that is based on a broad theoretical understanding of culture and ethnicity. Generic cultural competence abstracts general principles from specific examples of cultural differences. The core of generic competence resides in clinicians' understanding of their own cultural background and assumptions, some of which are related to ethnicity and religion and many of which derive from professional training and the context of practice. Appreciating the wide range of cultural variation in gender roles, family structures, developmental trajectories, explanations of health and illness, and responses to adversity allows the clinician to ask appropriate questions about areas that would otherwise be taken for granted. The culturally competent clinician has a keen sense of what he or she does not know and a solid respect for difference. While empathy and respectful interest allow the clinician gradually to come to know another's world, the clinician must tolerate the ambiguity and uncertainty that comes with not knowing. In the end, patients are the experts on their own experiential worlds, and cultural context must be reconstructed simultaneously from the inside out (through the patient's experience) and from the outside in (through an appreciation of the social matrix in which the patient is embedded).

The wide range of specific and generic skills needed for competent intercultural work means that most clinicians will find it helpful to work in multidisciplinary teams that contain cultural diversity that reflects the patient population. A variety of models for such teamwork have been developed.

Working with Interpreters and Culture-Brokers

A key skill that has not been addressed in many training programs concerns how to work with interpreters (Table 3.2). In the absence of familiarity with this technique and quality assurance standards insisting on appropriate use of interpreters, many clinicians simply try to avoid the situation, relying on patients' sometimes limited command of the clinician's language. This is unfortunate and may lead to errors in diagnosis and management as well as the failure to engage and help many patients.

There are several models of working with interpreters. Medical interpreters have adopted a code of ethics and model of working that owes much to forensic and political interpreting. Their goal is to provide accurate, complete, and literal translation of the statements of patient and physician. This model tends to portray the interpreter as

Table 3.2 Guidelines for Working with Interpreters and Culture-Brokers

Before the interview

- Explain the goals of the interview to the interpreter.
- Clarify the roles of interpreter and clinician, and the conduct of the interview.
- Discuss the interpreter's social position in country of origin and local community as it may influence the relationship with the patient.
- Explain the need for literal translation in the Mental Status Examination (e.g., to ascertain thought disorder, emotional range and appropriateness, and suicidality).
- Ask for feedback when something is hard to translate.
- Discuss etiquette and cultural expectations.

After the interview

- Debrief the interpreter to address any of their own emotional reactions and concerns.
- Discuss the process of the interview, any significant communication that was not translated, including paralanguage.
- Assess the patient's degree of openness or disclosure.
- Consider translation difficulties, misunderstandings.
- Plan future interviews.
- Work with the same interpreter/culture-broker for the same case whenever possible.

providing a transparent window or conduit of communication between clinician and patient. In this approach, the clinician addresses the patient directly as though the interpreter is not present. The interpreter may speak in the first person for the patient and for the clinician alternately. The model assumes that it is possible to achieve complete and accurate translation of messages in both directions and treats the interpersonal triad of doctor–interpreter–patient as if it were a dyad. To do so assumes that the interpreter does not have an independent relationship with patient or clinician. Of course, this is certainly not the case in any clinical encounter that goes on for a time or involves repeated meetings. Indeed, at the level of transference, it is never the case because the mere presence of another person immediately evokes distinctive thoughts, feelings, and fantasies. Then too, the presence of the interpreter inevitably changes a dyad into a triadic social system with its own complex interpersonal dynamics. These dynamics are complicated by the ethnocultural background of the interpreter and his or her own cultural assumptions.

The very idea of literal translation is also problematic. Across languages, words and phrases with similar denotation often have different sets of connotations. Every translation, therefore, is an interpretation that emphasizes some potential meanings while muting or eliding others. Interpreters tend to smooth out fragmentary, incomplete, or incoherent statements and so may mask thought disorder or other idiosyncrasies of speech with diagnostic relevance. The clinician needs to understand the choice of alternatives made by the interpreter in order to appreciate the connotations of the patient's words and to convey his or her own nuanced meanings. These requirements place much higher demands on interpreting in a mental health setting than in other medical or legal settings.

A slightly different model views the interpreter as a "go-between". In this approach, the interpreter takes turns interacting with clinician and patient to clarify what is being said and to find a means of conveying it. This model acknowledges the interpreter as an active intermediary and allows the interpreter some autonomy. The sequential dyadic interaction puts greater time and distance between clinician and patient. This demands that the interpreter have a high degree of clinical knowledge and interpersonal skill, which is possible when the interpreter has been trained as a clinician. Taking this autonomy further, the interpreter may be viewed as a cotherapist. In this approach, the interpreter with clinical skills develops his or her own working alliance with the patient. The interpreter may respond independently to the patient and initiate interventions. This sometimes happens because of language barriers, when patients may contact the interpreter to ask for help with practical issues.

Given the complexities of interpreting, we prefer to view the interpreter as a culture-broker who works to provide both the patient and the clinician with the cultural context needed to understand each other's meanings. To do this, the interpreter must understand something of the perspectives, cultural background, and social positions of both patient and clinician and appreciate the goals of the clinical task. Based on this knowledge, the culture-broker can enhance patient and clinician understanding of each other and can help negotiate compromises when there are widely divergent understandings of a problem and its solutions.

Despite increasing recognition of the importance of adequate interpretation, many clinicians or institutions use lay interpreters who are directly available at no cost, usually family members (even children) or other workers within the institution. Except in emergency situations, this practice should be avoided because it exerts a strong censorship on what may be disclosed in the encounter and because it may damage relationships that are very important to the patient by transgressing certain social and familial taboos.

Both interpreters and culture-brokers need training to perform competently, and clinicians need training, in turn, to work with these allied professionals. The clinician must take a systemic approach, understanding the other people in the room as part of an interactional system. Clinicians must also understand the interpreter's position in the larger community. Some of this training can go on when clinicians have an opportunity to work repeatedly with the same interpreters, who thus become part of a treatment team (Clinical Vignette 9).

Clinical Vignette 9

A 42-year-old man from the Congo is referred for psychiatric consultation because of concern that he is depressed following chemotherapy for leukemia. The patient lies in bed staring out the window and complaining of poor appetite, headache, and fatigue. At first, he says little to the Euro-Canadian interviewer. After a few minutes of stilted conversation, the culture-broker, a psychologist from central Africa, stands at the foot of the bed and delivers a lecture full of exhortations to the patient. He explains that the doctor has come to help, urges the patient to cooperate with the doctor, and insists that he must try to get better. After this intervention, the patient speaks more openly, clarifying that his fatigue and poor appetite are not due to depression or the lingering effects of chemotherapy but stem from the absence of appropriate African foods in his diet and the fear that he will die an improper death, far from home. His symptoms improve markedly once suitable food is arranged by contacting supportive members of his cultural community.

Conclusion: The Limits of Culture

The cultural formulation and the basic strategies of cultural competence represent useful initial approaches to exploring clinically relevant dimensions of patients' cultural backgrounds. However, to apply these tools successfully, the clinician must avoid some biases implicit in psychiatric assessment and in the concept of culture itself.

Psychiatric diagnosis tends to be individual-centered, locating problems inside the individual, in their psychology, or neurophysiology. Cultural psychiatry, in agreement with family theory and therapy, recognizes that many problems are systemic and reside in interpersonal interactions or social contexts.

In the cultural formulation, culture tends to appear as something distinctive of patients who come from ethnocultural minorities, migrants, or indigenous peoples. The clinician too has a culture that is distinctive from the patients' point of view. Indeed, culture also constitutes the larger social matrix in which the clinical encounter is embedded. The cultural critique of psychiatric theory and practice are important correctives to this view of culture as something only possessed by the "other".

Talk of culture tends to reify and essentialize it as a fixed set of traits or characteristics shared by all members of a group. However, there is enormous diversity and individual variation within any cultural group, and many divergent perspectives. The integrated whole of culture then appears to be a fiction or idealization. Contemporary anthropologists have argued for entirely dispensing with the notion of culture or else viewing it as an abstraction for a shifting set of perspectives, discourses, and resources used by individuals and groups to construct and position socially viable selves. This perspective recognizes that cultures are flexible frameworks that provide both opportunities and constraints but do not wholly determine the trajectories of individual lives.

With these caveats in mind, the clinician can apply the cultural formulation by approaching each case as unique, with a focus on the social and cultural context of the behavior and experience of the identified patient and his or her family. Cultural competence involves using one's knowledge of culture, language, and etiquette as modes of inquiry rather than as a priori answers to the dilemmas of a specific case. With the help of cultural experts, the clinician can appreciate the range of variation in a cultural group and its significance for individuals and the community. In this way, it is possible to recognize when culture is a camouflage for problems at other levels and when it is constitutive of problems itself. In assessment, the aim is to formulate cultural dynamics as part of a comprehensive process model of pathology. This can then be used to design interventions to address the most flexible or accessible level of the individual, family, or social system. Whenever possible, clinical interventions should mobilize and work with the family and ethnocultural community, who will have their own strategies and resources for problem solving and coping with adversity.

Cultural competence is based on respect for and interest in difference. It requires that clinicians become familiar with and comfortable talking about cultural differences rather than attempting to "treat everyone the same" in a misguided sense of "color blindness" or "neutrality"; lack of recognition of important differences results in ethnocentrism, seeing the world strictly from one's own cultural point of view. Instead, the clinician must learn to decenter, to encounter the other on a more equal footing, which allows some questioning of cultural assumptions relevant to psychiatric practice.

Mainstream care cannot respond adequately to the needs of a diverse population unless it gives explicit attention to cultural issues. The ethnocultural diversity of mental health professionals represents an invaluable resource. Training programs must recognize this and make it safe for clinicians to explore their own ethnocultural background and assumptions as a path to more sensitive and responsive work with others.

References

American Psychiatric Association (1994) *Diagnostic and Statistical Manual of Mental Disorders*, 4th edn. American Psychiatric Association, Washington, DC, pp. 843–849.

Kleinman A, Das V and Lock M (eds) (1997) *Social Suffering*. University of California Press, Berkeley.

References

CHAPTER

4 The Psychiatric Interview: Settings and Techniques

The interview is the principal means of assessment in clinical psychiatry. Despite major advances in neuroimaging and neurochemistry, there are no laboratory procedures as informative as observing, listening to, and interacting with the patient, and none as yet are more than supplementary to the information gathered by the psychiatric interview. This chapter deals with the interview as a means of assessing the patient and developing an initial treatment plan in clinical situations.

Psychiatric interviews are analogous to the history and physical examination in a general medical assessment; they systematically survey subjective and objective aspects of illness, and generate a differential diagnosis and plan for further evaluation and treatment. They differ from other medical interviews in the wide range of biological and psychosocial data that they must take into account, and in their attention to the emotional reactions of the patient and the process of interaction between the patient and interviewer. The nature of the interaction is informative diagnostically and is a means of building rapport and eliciting the patient's cooperation.

The style and content of a psychiatric interview are necessarily shaped by the interviewer's theory of psychopathology. Thus, a biological theory of illness leads to an emphasis on signs, symptoms, and course of illness; a psychodynamic theory dictates a focus on motivations, attitudes, feelings, and personal interactions; a behavioral viewpoint looks at antecedents and consequences of symptoms or maladaptive behaviors. In past times, when these and other theories competed for theoretical primacy, an interviewer might have viewed exploration from a particular single perspective as adequate. However, modern psychiatry views these perspectives as complementary rather than mutually exclusive, and recognizes the contributions of biological, intrapsychic, social, and environmental factors to human behavior and its disorders. The interviewer, therefore, faces the task of understanding each of these dimensions, adequately surveying them in the interview, and making informed judgments about their relative importance and treatment implications.

The written psychiatric database, the mental organization that the interviewer maintains during the interview, and the structure of the interview itself may differ

The Psychiatric Interview: Evaluation and Diagnosis, First Edition. Allan Tasman, Jerald Kay and Robert J. Ursano.

This chapter is based on Chapter 3 (Edward K. Silberman, Kenneth Certa, Abigail Kay) of *Psychiatry*, 3rd Edition.

considerably from one another. The written psychiatric database is an orderly exposition of information gathered in the interview, presented in a relatively fixed format.

The third structure is that of the interview itself. While guided by general principles of interviewing, this structure is the most flexible of the three, being determined not only by the purpose of the interview and the type of problem which the patient presents, but also by the patient's mode of communication and style of interaction with the interviewer. Thus, the interviewer must hold his or her own structure in mind while responding flexibly to the patient.

Goals of the Psychiatric Interview

The interviewer may be thought of as seeking the answers to several basic questions about the patient and the presenting problems. These questions provide the mental framework of the interview (although not its explicit form). They begin with triaging of patients into broad categories of type and severity, and progress to inquiry about details in each salient area. Table 4.1 lists the questions that the interview addresses and the implications of each for understanding and treating the patient. The answers to the questions in Table 4.1 are presented here in greater detail.

Does the Patient Have a Psychiatric Disorder?

This is the most basic question which the psychiatrist is called upon to answer, and determines whether or not there is any need for further psychiatric assessment or treatment.

How Severe Is the Illness?

The answer to this question determines the necessary level of treatment, ranging from hospitalization with close observation to infrequent outpatient visits. The main determinants of severity are dangerousness to self and others and impairment in ability to care for oneself and function in social and occupational roles.

What Is the Diagnosis?

In psychiatry, as in the rest of medicine, descriptive information about signs, symptoms, and course over time is used to assign a diagnosis to the presenting problem. Not all psychiatric diagnoses have similarly studied validity, but most convey the field's present knowledge of prognosis, comorbidity, treatment response, occurrence in family members, or associated biological or psychological findings. Even in the case of poorly understood entities, our present system of diagnosis using specific criteria maximizes uniformity in the description and naming of psychiatric disorders.

One important implication of diagnoses is whether there may be reduced plasticity of brain functioning due to anatomical or physiological abnormalities. Symptoms, deficits, and behaviors that stem from such abnormalities vary less in response to

Table 4.1 Issues to Be Addressed in a Psychiatric Assessment

Question	Implications
Does the patient have a psychiatric disorder?	Need for treatment
How severe is the disorder?	Need for hospitalization Need for structure or assistance in daily life Ability to function in major life roles
Are there abnormalities of brain function?	Degree of dysfunction of major mental processes such as perception, cognition, communication, regulation of mood and affect Responsivity of symptoms to environmental and motivation features Responsivity of symptoms to biological treatment
What is the diagnosis?	Description of the illness prognosis and treatment response
What is the patient's baseline level of functioning?	Determination of onset of illness State vs. trait pathology Goals for treatment Capacity for treatment
What environmental issues contribute to the disorder?	Prediction of conditions that may trigger future episodes of illness Need for focus on precipitating stressors Prevention of future episodes through amelioration of environmental stressors and/or increased environmental/social support
What biological factors contribute to the disorder?	Need for biological therapy Place of biological factors in explanation of illness presented to the patient Focus on biological factors as part of ongoing therapy
What psychological factors contribute to the disorder?	Responsivity of the symptoms to motivational, interpersonal, reinforcement factors Need to deal with psychological or interpersonal issues in therapy
What is the patient's motivation and capacity for treatment?	Decision to treat Choice of treatment

environmental and motivational factors than those behaviors that arise in the context of normal brain function. For example, mood swings in a patient with bipolar disorder, a condition for which there is strong evidence of a biological–genetic etiology, typically recur at regular time intervals, often independently of the patient's life situation. By contrast, mood swings in a patient with narcissistic personality disorder are much more likely to be triggered by interactions with other people. Furthermore, when brain function is impaired, biological treatments are more likely to be necessary, and verbal, interpersonal, or environmental interventions are less likely to be sufficient. Thus, the likelihood of altered brain function has major implications for understanding and treating the patient's problems.

Although the question of brain abnormalities is basic to psychiatric triaging, we do not yet have a clear-cut biological etiology for any disorder outside of those historically classified as "organic". Standard laboratory studies (such as brain imaging or electroencephalography) are not generally diagnostic of psychopathology; however, there is research-based evidence of altered brain function in many psychiatric disorders. Table 4.2 presents an overview of the current state of knowledge of brain abnormalities in psychiatric disorders, along with known responses to biological and psychosocial treatments.

What Is the Patient's Baseline Level of Functioning?

Determining what the patient has been like in his or her best or most usual state is a vital part of the assessment. This information allows the interviewer to gauge when the patient became ill, and how he or she is different when ill versus well. Environmental, biological, and psychological factors that contribute to low baseline levels of functioning may also predispose a patient to the development of psychiatric disorders. Thus, information about baseline functioning provides clues about the patient's areas of vulnerability to future illness as well as his or her capacity to benefit from treatment. It is also an important guide to realistic goals and expectations for such treatment. Table 4.3 lists major components of functioning with examples of elements of each.

What Environmental Factors Contribute to the Disorder?

Environmental contributions to the presenting problem are factors external to the patient. They may be acute events that precipitate illness, or longstanding factors that increase general vulnerability. Longstanding environmental stressors may predispose the patient to the development of illness and may also worsen the outlook for recovery.

It is important to identify adverse environmental influences that can be modified, and to help the patient or family make necessary changes. For example, a patient with recurrent paranoid psychosis needed yearly hospitalization as long as she worked in an office with many other people. However, she no longer suffered severe relapses when she was helped to find work that she could do in her own home. However, even irreversible precipitants, such as death of a loved one, must be identified and dealt with in the treatment plan.

What Biological Factors Contribute to the Disorder?

Biological factors may contribute to psychiatric disorders directly by their effects on the central nervous system and indirectly through the effects of pain, disability, or social

Table 4.2 Brain Dysfunction in Psychiatric Disorders

Disorder	Evidence for Brain Dysfunction	Response to Biological Treatments	Response to Psychosocial Treatments
Delirium, dementia, amnestic and cognitive disorders (Leigh and Reiser, 1992; Lipowski, 1984; Lishman, 1978; Popkin, 1994)	Well established	Reversible causes respond to appropriate treatment, neuroleptics, anxiolytics, antidepressants, lithium, and anticonvulsants. Beta-blockers may be helpful	Environmental support and supportive psychotherapy may be helpful
Schizophrenia (Bellack and Mueser, 1993; Carpenter and Buchanan, 1994; Davis, 1975; Kotrla and Weinberger, 1995; Sensky *et al.*, 2000)	Strong evidence	Most respond to antipsychotics; antidepressants, mood stabilizers, and anxiolytics may be helpful adjunctively	Environmental support, supportive psychotherapy, cognitive–behavioral therapy, family therapy, and skills training are helpful
Delusional disorder (Maber, 1992; Manschreck, 1996)	Little evidence – few studies	Poor to fair response to psychotics	Poor response to psychotherapy
Schizoaffective disorder (Keck *et al.*, 1996; Kendler, 1991; Winokur *et al.*, 1996)	Evidence for relationship to schizophrenia and mood disorders	Most respond to combinations of antipsychotics, antidepressants, mood stabilizers, carbamazepine, electroconvulsive therapy (ECT)	Not well established. Similar range of treatments as for schizophrenia may be helpful
Brief psychotic disorder (Jorgensen *et al.*, 1996; Susser *et al.*, 1995)	Little evidence – few studies	Not well established	Environmental support and supportive psychotherapy may be helpful
Bipolar disorder (Goodwin and Jamison, 1990; Janowsky *et al.*, 1974; Tsuang and Faraone, 1990)	Strong evidence	Most respond to lithium, antidepressants, anticonvulsants, neuroleptics, or ECT	Supportive and educative psychotherapy and family therapy may be helpful

(*Continued*)

Table 4.2 *(Cont'd)*

Disorder	Evidence for Brain Dysfunction	Response to Biological Treatments	Response to Psychosocial Treatments
Major depressive disorder (Elkin *et al.*, 1989; Siever and Davis, 1985; Thase and Howland, 1995)	Evidence suggestive – considerable heterogeneity	Often responds to antidepressants or ECT	Less severe cases respond to cognitive, interpersonal, and psychodynamic psychotherapy
Panic disorder (Barlow, 1988; Barlow *et al.*, 2000; Goddard and Charney, 1997; Milrod *et al.*, 2000)	Evidence suggestive	Most respond to anxiolytics or antidepressants	Variable. Cognitive–behavioral therapy more effective than psychodynamic
Generalized anxiety disorder (Blazer *et al.*, 1991)	Little evidence	Variable. Anxiolytics may be helpful	Variable. Psychodynamic or cognitive–behavioral psychotherapies are often helpful
Simple phobia (Fyer *et al.*, 1990; Marks, 1987)	Little evidence	Medications not usually helpful	Most respond to behavioral therapy
Posttraumatic stress disorder (Heim *et al.*, 2000; Katz *et al.*, 1996; Marks *et al.*, 1998)	Evidence suggestive	Variable. Antidepressants and mood stabilizers may be helpful	Psychotherapy with exploratory, supportive, and behavioral features usually helpful
Obsessive–compulsive disorder (Abramowitz, 1997; Baxter, 1992; Insel, 1992)	Evidence suggestive	Most respond to selective serotonin reuptake inhibitors	Rituals but not obsessive thoughts respond to behavioral therapy
Somatization disorder (Cloninger *et al.*, 1986; Min and Lee, 1997)	Preliminary evidence	Poor. Medication for comorbid depression or anxiety may help	Poor. Supportive psychotherapy may help

Conversion disorder (Ford and Foulks, 1985; Lazare, 1981)	None known	Amytal interview may help; otherwise not indicated	Most respond to psychotherapy with exploratory, expressive, and behavioral features. May remit spontaneously
Hypochondriasis (Ford, 1995; Kellner, 1987)	None known	No direct response. Medications may help for treatment of comorbid depression and anxiety	Variable. Supportive–educative psychotherapy may be helpful
Dissociative disorders (Brenner and Marmer, 1998; Kluft and Fine, 1993)	None known	No direct response. Medications may help for treatment of comorbid depression and anxiety	Variable. Many respond to expressive–exploratory psychotherapy
Alcoholism (Merlett, 1998; Prescott and Kendler, 1999)	Strong evidence in subgroups	No well-demonstrated direct effects. Opiate antagonists may be helpful	Group and individual psychotherapies most common treatment modalities. Response variable, relapse high
Psychoactive substance use disorders (Banmohl and Jaffe, 1995; Nesse and Berridge, 1997)	Little evidence – some subgroups	No well-demonstrated direct effects	Group and individual psychotherapies most common treatment modalities. Response variable, relapse high
Sexual disorder (LoPiccolo, 1985; Marshall and Barbaree, 1990)	May be due to metabolic disorders; otherwise little evidence	Medications for underlying medical conditions may be necessary. Antiandrogens or serotonergic antidepressants may be helpful for paraphilias	Sexual dysfunctions often respond to behavior therapy. Couples therapy or exploratory therapy may also be helpful
Eating disorders (Halmi, 1992; Johnson and Connors, 1987)	Evidence suggestive	Antidepressants may help ameliorate symptoms	Expressive exploration, family, and behavioral therapy often helpful

(*Continued*)

Table 4.2 *(Cont'd)*

Disorder	Evidence for Brain Dysfunction	Response to Biological Treatments	Response to Psychosocial Treatments
Adjustment disorders (Andreasen and Hoevk, 1982; Greenberg *et al.*, 1995)	None known	Medications may alleviate symptoms of anxiety or depression	Supportive psychotherapy often helpful
Personality disorders: Cluster A (Kendler *et al.*, 1984; Siever *et al.*, 1991)	Evidence for relationship of schizotypal personality to schizophrenia; otherwise none known	Schizotypal patients may improve on antipsychotic medication; otherwise not indicated	Poor. Supportive psychotherapy may help
Personality disorders: Cluster B (Bateman and Fonagy, 2001; Clarkin *et al.*, 2007; Coccaro and Kavoussi, 1997; Tarnepolsky and Berlowitz, 1987; Zuckerman, 1996)	Evidence suggestive for antisocial and borderline personalities; otherwise none known	Antidepressants, antipsychotics, mood stabilizers may help for borderline personality; otherwise not indicated	Poor in antisocial personality. Variable in borderline, narcissistic, and histrionic personalities
Personality disorders: Cluster C (Cloninger, 1987; Cloninger *et al.*, 1993; Millon, 1996; Svartberg *et al.*, 2004)	None known	No direct response. Medications may help with comorbid anxiety, depression	Psychodynamic psychotherapy and cognitive behavior therapy

Table 4.3 Assessment of Baseline Functioning

Component	Examples
Level of symptoms	Depression Anxiety, obsessions, and compulsions Delusion Hallucinations
Interpersonal relations	Sexual relationships and marriage Quality and longevity of friendships Capacity for intimacy and commitment
Work adjustment	Employment history Level of responsibility Functioning in nonpaid roles, e.g., homemaker, parent Satisfaction with work life
Leisure activities	Hobbies and interests Group and social activities Travel Ability to take pleasure in nonwork activities
Ego functions	Talents, skills, intelligence Ability to cope; reality testing Control over affects and behaviors Ability to formulate and carry through plans Stable sense of self and others Capacity for self-observation

stigma. Thus, biological factors must be assessed through both the psychiatric history and diagnosis, and the general medical history.

Biological factors affecting the central nervous system may be genetic, prenatal, perinatal, or postnatal. Conditions such as maternal substance abuse or intrauterine infections may affect fetal brain development; birth complications may cause cerebral hypoxia with resultant brain damage. In postnatal life, the entire range of diseases that affect the brain may alter mental function and behavior, as may exposure to toxins at work, in the environment, and through substance abuse. In addition, medical conditions that do not directly affect brain functioning may have profound effects on the patient's state of mind and behavior (Clinical Vignettes 1, 2 and 3).

Biological factors may both predispose to and precipitate episodes of illness. Thus, a patient with a genetic vulnerability to schizophrenic illness may have an episode of acute psychosis precipitated by heavy cocaine use. Similarly, a patient with borderline low intellectual capacity due to hypoxia at birth may have marginal ability to care for herself. An accident resulting in a fractured arm might overwhelm this person's coping capacity and precipitate a severe adjustment disorder.

Clinical Vignette 1

A 30-year-old married woman suffers from chronic low mood and lack of enjoyment of life. She is highly dependent on her husband for practical and emotional support, although she frequently flies into rages at him, feeling that he is cold and uncaring. She has had a series of secretarial jobs which she begins enthusiastically, but soon comes to feel that her employers are highly critical and belittling, whereupon she resigns. Her friendships are limited to people with whom she can have very special, exclusive relationships. She deals poorly with change or loss, which frequently trigger episodes of acute dysfunction. When a friend is not sufficiently available to her, she feels betrayed and worthless, her mood plummets, she becomes lethargic, has eating binges, and is unable to work or pursue her usual routine for up to weeks at a time.

Clinical Vignette 2

A patient functions well in a responsible job and has had a long-standing, stable marriage. However, he is driven by the need to be liked and accepted by all who know him, and has a deep-seated, but not conscious, belief that he must continually fulfill the wishes of others in order to accomplish this. At the same time, he has a chronic feeling of powerlessness and an unarticulated wish to be able to say no. At times of increased demands by family members or coworkers, he develops flu-like symptoms and stays home from work "recuperating", relieved of responsibility for fulfilling the expectations of others.

Clinical Vignette 3

A young woman became acutely depressed upon receiving her acceptance to medical school. She was the oldest of four children and had been expected to assume a major caretaking role with her younger siblings. Her mother, a busy physician, wished for her daughter to have a similar career. To the patient, entering medical school meant accepting a lifelong role as a caretaker and forever relinquishing her own wishes to be taken care of.

What Psychological Factors Contribute to the Disorder?

Psychological factors are mental traits that the patient brings to life situations. While they interact with social and environmental factors, they are intrinsic to the individual, and not readily changed by outside influences.

Psychological factors predisposing to illness include both general and focal deficits in coping adaptability. General deficits encompass the entire range of ego functioning, including poor reality testing, rigid or maladaptive psychological defense mechanisms, low ability to tolerate and contain affects, impulsivity, poorly formed or unstable sense of self, low self-esteem and hostile, distant, or dependent relationships with others. Patients with such deficits generally meet diagnostic criteria for one or more personality disorders and are at increased risk for episodes of acute psychiatric illness. An example of general deficits in psychological functioning is illustrated by the following case.

Focal psychological issues may also contribute to mental disorders. These issues, which typically involve conflicts between opposing motivations, may affect the patient in certain specific areas of function or life situations, leaving other broad areas of function intact (Nemiah, 1961). Such conflicts are most likely to cause maladaptive behaviors or symptoms when the patient is not clearly aware of them.

The meaning of an event in the context of the patient's life course is another focal issue that may contribute to illness.

What Is the Patient's Motivation and Capacity for Treatment?

Whatever the physician's view of the presenting problem, the patient's wishes and capacities are an important determinant of treatment choice. Some patients seek relief of symptoms; some wish to change their behavior or the nature of their relationships; some want to understand themselves better. Patients may wish to talk or to receive medication or instructions.

The patient's capacity for treatment must also be considered in the treatment plan. For example, a patient with schizophrenia may agree to medication but be too disorganized to take it reliably without help.

The Psychiatric Database

The body of information to be gathered from the interview may be termed "the psychiatric database" (Table 4.2, Table 4.3, and Table 4.4). It is a variable set of data: either very specific or general, mainly limited to the present state or focused on early life, dominated by neurological questions or inquiry into relationships. To avoid setting the impossible task of learning everything about every patient, one must consider certain factors that modify the required database.

Whose questions are to be answered – the patient's concern about himself or herself, a family or friend's concern about him or her, another physician's diagnostic dilemma, a civil authority's need to safeguard the public, or a research protocol requirement? Who will have access to the data gathered and under what circumstances? What is the setting of the interview? Is the interview to be the first session of a psychotherapy regimen, or is it a one time only evaluation? What is the nature of the pathology? For example, negative responses regarding the presence of major psychotic symptoms, coupled with a history of good occupational function, will generally preclude a detailed inventory of psychotic features. A missed orientation or memory question will require careful cognitive testing. Patients with personality disorder symptoms warrant careful attention to the history of significant relationships (Nurnberg *et al.*, 1991), work history, and the feelings evoked in the interviewer during the

Table 4.4 Core Database

Identifying Data	Chief Complaint	History of Present Illness
Name	**Reason for Consultation**	**Major Symptoms**
Age/date of birth; next of kin		Time course Stressors Change in functioning Current medical problems and treatment
Past psychiatric history	Past medical history	Family history
Any previous psychiatric treatment	Ever hospitalized Surgery Medications	Psychiatric illness
History of suicide attempts		
Functioning problems secondary to psychiatric symptoms Alcohol/drug abuse		
Personal history	Mental status	
Educational level Ever married/committed relationship	Appearance Attitude Affect Behavior	
Work history Means of support Living situation Thought process Thought content Perception Cognition Insight Judgment	Speech	

evaluation process. The database should be expanded in areas of diagnostic concern to support or rule out particular syndromes. The amount and nature of the data obtained is also, of necessity, limited by the patient's ability to communicate and his or her cooperativeness.

Database Components

Identifying Data

This information establishes the patient's identity, especially for the purpose of obtaining past history from other contacts, when necessary, as well as fixing his or her position in society. The patient's name should be recorded, along with any nickname or alternative names he or she may have been known by in the past. This is important for women who might have been treated previously under a maiden name, or a patient who has had legal entanglements and so has adopted aliases.

Date of birth, or at least age, and race are other essential parts of every person's database. People of white, black (or African-American), Asian, Native American, and other origins are generally accepted. The additional modifier of ethnicity, especially Hispanic/non-Hispanic, is becoming more widely used. If a patient is a member of a particular subculture based on ethnicity, country of origin, or religious affiliation, it may be noted here.

A traditional part of the identifying data is a reference to the patient's civil status: single, married, separated, divorced, or widowed. The patient's social security number (or other national ID number) can be a very useful bit of data when seeking information from other institutions.

In most cases, it is assumed that the informant (supplier of the history) is the patient. If other sources are used, and especially if the patient is not the primary informant, this should be noted at the beginning of the database.

Chief Complaint

The chief complaint is the patient's responses to the question, "What brings you to see me/to the hospital today?" or some variant thereof. It is usually quoted verbatim, placed within quotation marks, and should be no more than one or two sentences.

Even if the patient is very disorganized or hostile, quoting his response can give an immediate sense of where the patient is as the interview begins. If the patient responds with an expletive, or a totally irrelevant remark, the reader of the database is immediately informed about how the rest of the information may be distorted. In such cases, or if the patient gives no response, a brief statement of how the patient came to be evaluated should be made and enclosed in parentheses.

History of the Present Illness

Minimum Essential Database

The present illness history should begin with a brief description of the major symptoms that brought the patient to psychiatric attention. The most troubling symptoms should be detailed initially; later, a more thorough review will be stated. As a minimum, the approximate time since the patient was last at his or her baseline level of functioning, and in what way he or she is different from that now, should be described, and any known stressors, the sequence of symptom development, and the beneficial or deleterious effects of interventions included.

How far back in a patient's history to go, especially when he or she has chronic psychiatric illness, is sometimes problematic. In patients who have required repeated hospitalization, a summary of events since last discharge (if within 6 months) or last stable baseline is indicated. It is rare that more than 6 months of history be included in the history of the present illness, and detailed history is more commonly given on the past month.

Expanded Database

A more expanded description of the history of the present illness would include events in a patient's life at the onset of symptoms, as well as exactly how the symptoms have affected the patient's occupational functioning and important relationships. Any concurrent medical illness symptoms, medication usage (and particularly changes), alterations in the sleep–wake cycle, appetite disturbances, and eating patterns should be noted; significant negative findings should also be remarked upon.

Past Psychiatric History

Minimum Essential Database

Most of the major psychiatric illnesses are chronic in nature. For this reason, often patients have had previous episodes of illness with or without treatment. New onset of symptoms, without any previous psychiatric history, becomes increasingly important with advancing age in terms of diagnostic categories to be considered. At a minimum, the presence or absence of past psychiatric symptomatology should be recorded, along with psychiatric interventions taken and the result of such interventions. An explicit statement about past suicide and homicide attempts should be included.

Expanded Database

A more detailed history would include names and places of psychiatric treatment, dosages of medications used, and time course of response. The type of psychotherapy, the patient's feelings about former therapists, his or her compliance with treatment, as well as circumstances of termination are also important. Note what the patient has learned about the biological and psychological factors predisposing him or her to illness, and whether there were precipitating events.

Past Medical History

Minimum Essential Database

In any clinical assessment, it is important to know how a patient's general health status has been. In particular, any current medical illness and treatment should be noted along with any major past illness requiring hospitalization.

Expanded Database

An expanded database could well include significant childhood illnesses, how these were handled by the patient and his or her family, and therefore the degree to which the patient was able to develop a sense of comfort and security about his or her physical well-being. Illnesses later in life should be assessed for the degree of regression produced. The amount of time a patient has had to take off work, how well he or she was able to follow a regimen of medical care, his or her relationship with the family physician or treating specialist can all be useful in predicting future response to treatment. A careful past medical history can also at times bring to light a suicide attempt, substance abuse, or dangerously careless behavior, which might not be obtained any other way.

Family History

Minimum Essential Database

Given the evidence for familial, genetic factors in so many psychiatric conditions, noting the presence of mental illness in biological relatives of the patient is necessary. It is important to specify during questioning the degree of family to be considered – usually to the second degree: aunts, uncles, cousins, and grandparents, as well as parents, siblings, and children.

Expanded Database

A history of familial medical illness is a useful part of an expanded database. A genogram (pedigree), including known family members with dates and causes of death and other known chronic illnesses is helpful. Questioning about causes of death will also occasionally bring out hidden psychiatric illness, for example, sudden, unexpected deaths, which were likely suicides or illness secondary to substance abuse.

Personal History

Minimum Essential Database

Recording the story of a person's life can be a daunting undertaking and is often where a database can expand dramatically. As a minimum, this part of the history should include where a patient was born and raised, and in what circumstances – intact family, number of siblings, and degree of material comfort. Note how far the patient went in school, how he or she did there, and what his or her occupational functioning has been. If he or she is not working, why not? Has the patient ever been involved in criminal activity, and with what consequences? Has the patient ever married or been involved in a committed relationship? Are there any children? What is his or her current source of support? Does he or she live alone or with someone? Has he or she ever used alcohol or other drugs to excess, and is there current use? Has he or she ever been physically or sexually abused or been the victim of some other trauma?

Expanded Database

An expanded database can include a great deal of material beginning even prior to the patient's conception. What follows is an outline of the kind of data that may be gathered, along with an organizational framework.

Family of Origin

Were parents married or in committed relationships?
Personality and significant events in life of mother, father, or other significant caregiver.
Siblings: number? their ages, significant life events, personality, relationship to patient.
Who else shared the household with the family?

Prenatal and Perinatal

Was the pregnancy planned? Quality of prenatal care; mother's and father's response to pregnancy.
Illness, medication or substance abuse, smoking, trauma during pregnancy; labor – induced or spontaneous?
Weeks gestation, difficulty of delivery, vaginal or Caesarean section.
Presence of jaundice at birth, birth weight, Apgar score.
Baby went home with mother or stayed on in hospital.

Early Childhood

Developmental milestones: smiling, sitting, standing, walking, talking, type of feeding – food allergies or intolerance.
Consistency of caregiving: interruptions by illness, birth of siblings.
Reaction to weaning, toilet-training, maternal separation.
Earliest memories: problematic behavior (tantrums, bedwetting, hair-pulling, or nail-biting).
Temperament (shy, overactive, outgoing, fussy).
Sleep problems: insomnia, nightmares, enuresis, parasomnias.

Later Childhood

Early school experiences: evidence of separation anxiety.
Behavioral problems at home or school: firesetting, bedwetting, aggressive toward others, cruelty to animals, nightmares.
Developmental milestones: learning to read, write.
Relationships with other children and family: any loss or trauma.
Reaction to illness.

Adolescence

School performance: ever in special classes?
Athletic abilities and participation in sports.
Evidence of gender identity concerns: overly "feminine" or "masculine" in appearance/behavior, or perception by peers.

Ever run away? Able to be left alone and assume responsibility.
Age of onset of puberty (menarche or nocturnal emissions), reaction to puberty.

Identity

Sexual preference and gender identity, religious affiliation (same as parents?).
Career goals: ethnic identification.

Sexual History

Early sexual teaching: earliest sexual experiences, experience of being sexually abused, attitudes toward sexual behavior.
Dating history, precautions taken to prevent sexually transmitted diseases and/or pregnancy.
Episodes of impotence and reaction.
Masturbating patterns and fantasies.
Preoccupation with particular sexual practices, current sexual functioning, length of significant relationships, ages of partners.

Adulthood

Age at which left home, level of educational attainments.
Employment history, relationships with supervisors and peers at work, reasons for job change.
History of significant relationships including duration, typical roles in relationships, patterns of conflict: marital history, legal entanglements, and criminal history, both covert and detected, ever victim or perpetrator of violence.
Major medical illness as adult.
Participation in community affairs.
Financial status: own or rented home, stability of living situation.
Ever on disability or public assistance?
Current family structure, reaction to losses of missing members (parents, siblings), if applicable.
Substance abuse history.

Mental Status Examination

It can be helpful to conceptualize the recording of the Mental Status Examination (MSE) as a progression. One begins with a snapshot: what can be gained from a cursory visual exam, without any movement or interaction – appearance and affect. Next, motion is added: behavior. Then comes sound: the patient's speech, though initially only as sound. The ideas being expressed come next: the thought process and content, perception, cognition, insight, and judgment. Table 4.5 gives a summary of areas to be commented on, along with common terms.

At every level of the MSE, preference should be given for explicit description over jargon. Stating that a patient is delusional is less helpful than describing him as believing that his neighbors are pumping poisonous gases into his bedroom while he sleeps.

Table 4.5 Mental Status Examination

Appearance
Level of consciousness (alert, hypervigilant, somnolent, stuporous)
Dress (casual, appropriate for weather, eccentric, careless, disheveled)
Grooming (style of hair, degree of makeup, shaven/unshaven, clean, malodorous)
Idiosyncrasies – tattoos (professional or amateur), prominent scars, religious emblems

Attitude
Cooperative, hostile, evasive, threatening, obsequious

Affect
Range (restricted, expansive, blunted, flat)
Appropriateness to items discussed
Stability (labile, shallow)
Quality (silly, anxious)

Mood
Response to question: "How are you feeling/How's your mood been?"

Behavior
Psychomotor agitation or retardation

Speech
Rate (rapid, slowed, pressured, hard to interrupt)
Volume (loud, soft, monotone, highly inflected, or dramatic)
Quality (neologisms, fluent, idiosyncratic)

Thought process
Goal-directed, disorganized, loose associations, tangential, circumstantial, flight of ideas

Thought content
Major preoccupations, ideas of reference, delusions (grandiose, paranoid, bizarre; state exactly what it is the patient appears to believe)
Thought broadcasting, insertion, or withdrawal
Suicidal or homicidal ideation. Plan and intent to carry out ideas

Perception
Illusions and hallucinations – type (auditory, visual, olfactory, tactile, gustatory), evidence (patient spontaneous report, answer to interviewer question, observation of patient attending or responding to nonexistent external stimuli)
Patient's beliefs about hallucinatory phenomenon (do they seem to originate from the outside or inside, how many voices, what gender, talking to patient or to other voices, are they keeping up constant commentary on the patient)

Cognition
Orientation: time, place, person, situation
Memory: number of remembered objects, digit span, presidents backward, recent events

Concentration: serial 7s, *world* spelled backward
Abstraction: proverb interpretation – what would someone mean by "The grass is always greener on the other side of the fence" ("Get off my back")
Similarities: (How are these things alike – apple–orange, table–chair, eye–ear, praise–punishment?)
Computation: number of digits successfully added or subtracted, ability to calculate change
(How many quarters are in $1.50? If you bought a loaf of bread for 89 cents and gave the cashier a dollar, what change would you get back?)

Insight
Knows something is wrong, that he or she is ill, that illness is psychiatric; understands ways in which illness disrupts function

Judgment
Response to standard questions (If you found a sealed, addressed, stamped letter, what would you do? If you smelled smoke in a crowded theater?)
Evidence from behavior prior to and during interview (Was the patient caring for himself or herself properly, handling business affairs well? Does the behavior during the interview match his or her stated goals, e.g., if he or she wishes to be thought to be in control, is he or she keeping the voice down and movement in check?)

Conduct of the Interview: Factors That Affect the Interview

A skillful interview will not necessarily yield all the relevant information but will make the most of the opportunities in a clinical situation, given the limitations which both the patient and interviewer bring. Factors that influence the development of an alliance and the amount that can be learned in the interview include the following.

The Patient's Physical or Emotional Distress

Patients who are in acute distress either from physical discomfort or from emotional factors such as severe depression or anxiety will be limited in their motivation and ability to interact with the interviewer. The interviewer may be able to enhance communication by addressing the patient's discomfort in a supportive manner. However, he or she must also recognize times when the patient's discomfort necessitates a more limited interview.

The Cognitive Capacities of the Patient

Patients who are demented, retarded, disorganized, thought-disordered, amnesic, aphasic, or otherwise impaired in intellectual or cognitive capacity have biologically based deficits, which limit the amount of information they can convey.

The Emotionally Based Biases of the Patient

Patients bring to the interview a wide variety of preconceptions, expectations, and tendencies toward distortion, which influence how they view and relate to the interviewer. Such biases are commonly referred to as *transference* because they frequently can be understood as arising from interactions with important figures in childhood, such as parents, which serve as imprinted templates of perceptions of others. Transferential biases may be positive or negative. Thus, even before the start of the interview, one patient may be primed to view the doctor as a wise and kindly healer, while another will be predisposed to see him or her as an exploitative charlatan. Clearly, such biases affect the amount of openness and trust that the patient brings to the interview and the quality of information he or she provides.

The Emotionally Based Biases of the Interviewer

The interviewer, like the patient, may have feelings stirred up by the interaction. The interviewer's emotional reactions to the patient can be an invaluable asset in assessment if he or she can be conscious of them and reflect on their causes. For example, an interviewer finds himself or herself becoming increasingly annoyed at a highly polite patient. On reflection, he realizes that the politeness serves to rebuff his attempts to establish a warmer, more spontaneous relationship and is a manifestation of the patient's underlying hostile attitude.

When the interviewer is unable to monitor and examine his or her emotional reactions, they are more likely to impede rather than enhance understanding of the patient. This is most likely to happen when emotional reactions are driven more by the interviewer's own biases than by the patient's behavior. Such reactions are referred to as the interviewer's *countertransference*. The entire range of countertransferential interviewer attitudes toward the patient, from aversion to infatuation, might similarly bias judgment.

Situational Factors

Patients' attitudes toward the interview will be strongly influenced by the situation in which the consultation arises. Some patients decide for themselves that they need treatment, while others come reluctantly, under pressure from others. Patients who are being evaluated for disability or in connection with a lawsuit may feel a need to prove that they are ill, while those being evaluated for civil commitment or at the insistence of family members may need to prove that they are well. Similarly, a patient's past history of relationships with psychiatrists or with health professionals in general is likely to color his or her attitude toward the interviewer.

The interviewer may also be affected by situational factors. For example, pressure of time in a busy emergency service may influence the interviewer to omit important areas of inquiry and reach premature closure; the experience of a recent patient suicide may bias the interviewer toward overestimation of risk in someone with suicidal thoughts. As with countertransference reactions, it is important for the interviewer to minimize distortions due to situational factors by being as aware of them as possible.

Racial, Ethnic, and Cultural Factors

The degree of racial, ethnic, cultural, and socioeconomic similarity between the patient and interviewer can influence the course and outcome of the interview in many ways (see also Chapter 2). It may affect the level of rapport between patient and interviewer, the way both view the demands of the situation, the way they interpret each other's verbal and nonverbal communications, and the meaning the interviewer assigns to the patient's statements and behaviors. Not only racial or cultural prejudice but also well-intentioned ignorance can interfere with communication and accurate assessment.

Some cultures, for example, place a higher value on politeness and respect for authority than does Western culture. A patient from such a background might be reluctant to correct or disagree with the interviewer's statements even when they are erroneous. The interviewer might not suspect that he or she was hearing distorted information, or conversely, might see the patient as pathologically inhibited or unemotional. Many non-Western cultures place a higher value on family solidarity than on individuality. Pressing a patient from such a culture to report angry feelings toward family members might raise his or her anxiety, decrease rapport with the interviewer, and produce defensive distortions in the material.

General Features of Psychiatric Interviews

Setting

The ideal interview setting is one which provides a pleasant atmosphere and is reasonably comfortable, private, and free from outside distractions. Such a setting not only provides the physical necessities for an interview but conveys to the patient that he or she will be well cared for and safe. Providing such a setting may pose special problems in certain interviewing situations. For example, it may be necessary to interview highly agitated patients in the presence of security personnel; interviewers on medical–surgical units must pay special attention to the patient's comfort and privacy.

Verbal Communication

Verbal communication may be straightforward imparting of information: "Every year around November, I begin to lose interest in everything and my energy gets very low". However, patients may convey information indirectly through metaphor, or use words for noninformational purposes, such as to express or contain emotions or to create an impact on the interviewer.

In metaphorical language, one idea is represented by another with which it shares some features. For example, when asked how she gets along with her daughter-in-law, a woman replies: "I can never visit their house because she always likes to keep the thermostat down. It's never as warm as I need". Such a reply suggests that the woman may not feel "warmly" accepted and welcomed by her son's wife. Metaphor may also use the body to represent ideas or feelings. A man who proved to meet the diagnostic criteria for major depressive disorder described his mood as "OK" but complained that his life was being ruined by constant aching in his chest for which the doctors could find no cause. In this instance, the pain of depression was experienced and described metaphorically as a somatic symptom.

Language may be used to express emotions directly, but more often is used indirectly by influencing the process of the interview. Patients may shift topics, make off-hand remarks or jokes, ask questions, and compliment or belittle the interviewer as a way of expressing feelings. The process of the interview frequently expresses the patient's feelings about his or her immediate situation or interaction with the interviewer. For example, a woman being evaluated for depression and anxiety suddenly said: "I was just wondering doctor, do you have any children?" The further course of the interview revealed that she was terrified of being committed to a hospital and abandoned. The question was an attempt to establish whether the interviewer was a good parent and therefore safe as a caretaker for her.

Language may also be used in the service of psychological defense mechanisms to contain rather than express emotions. For example, a young man with generalized anxiety was asked whether he was sexually active. He replied by talking at length about how all the women he knew at college were either unappealing or attached to other men. Further discussion revealed that he developed severe symptoms of anxiety whenever he was with a woman to whom he felt sexually attracted. His initial reply represented an automatic, verbal mechanism (in this case, a rationalization) for keeping the anxiety out of awareness.

Another form of process communication is the use of language to make an impact on the interviewer. A statement such as "If you can't help me I'm going to kill myself" might convey suicidal intent, but may also serve to stir up feelings of concern and involvement in the interviewer. Similarly, the patient who says "Dr X really understood me, but he was much older and more experienced than you are" may be feeling vulnerable and ashamed, and unconsciously trying to induce similar feelings in the interviewer. When language is used in this way, the interviewer's subjective reaction may be the best clue to the underlying feelings and motivations of the patient.

Nonverbal Communication

Emotions and attitudes are communicated nonverbally through facial expressions, gestures, body position, and movements, interpersonal distance, dress and grooming, and speech. Some nonverbal communications such as gestures are almost always conscious and deliberate, while others often occur automatically outside one's awareness. The latter type are particularly important to observe during an interview because they may convey messages entirely separate from or even contradictory to what is being said.

The interviewer will automatically decode these signals but may ignore the message due to countertransference or social pressure from the patient. For example, a patient may say, "I feel very comfortable with you, doctor", but sit stiffly upright and maintain a rigidly fixed smile, conveying a strong nonverbal message of tension and mistrust. The nonverbal message may be missed if, for example, the interviewer has a strong need to be liked by the patient. Another patient denies angry feelings while sitting with a tightly clenched fist. The interviewer may unconsciously collude with the patient's need to avoid his anger by ignoring the body language.

As with any medical examination, observation of nonverbal behavior may provide important diagnostic information. For example, a leaden body posture may indicate depression, movements of the foot may arise from anxiety or tardive dyskinesia, and sudden turning of the head and eyes may suggest hallucinations.

Nonverbal communication proceeds in both directions, and the nonverbal messages of the interviewer are likely to have a considerable effect on the patient. Thus, the interviewer who sits back in his chair and looks down at his notes communicates less interest and involvement than one who sits upright and makes eye contact. Similarly, an interviewer who gives a weak handshake and sits behind a desk or far across the room from the patient will communicate a sense of distance, which may interfere with establishing rapport. It is important that the interviewer be aware of his or her own nonverbal messages and adapt them to the needs of the patient.

Listening and Observation

The interviewer must remain open to literal and metaphorical messages from the patient, to the impact the patient is trying to make and to the degree to which nonverbal communication complements or contradicts what is being said. Doing this optimally requires that the interviewer also be able to listen to his or her own mental processes throughout the interview, including both thoughts and emotional reactions. Listening of this kind depends upon having a certain level of comfort, confidence, and space to reflect, and may be very difficult when the patient is hostile, agitated, demanding, or putting pressure on the interviewer in any other way. With such patients, it may take many interviews to do enough good listening to gain an adequate understanding of the case.

Another important issue in listening is maintaining a proper balance between forming judgments and remaining open to new information and new hypotheses. On the one hand, one approaches the interview with knowledge of diagnostic classifications, psychological mechanisms, behavioral patterns, social forces, and other factors that shape one's understanding of the patient. The interviewer hears the material with an ear to fitting the information into these preformed patterns and categories. On the other hand, the interviewer must remain open to hearing and seeing things that extend or modify his or her judgments about the patient. At times, the interviewer may listen narrowly to confirm a hypothesis, while at others, he or she may listen more openly, with relatively little preconception. Thus, listening must be structured enough to generate a formulation but open enough to avoid premature judgments.

Attitude and Behavior of the Interviewer

The optimal attitude of the interviewer is one of interest, concern, and intention to help the patient. While the interviewer must be tactful and thoughtful about what he or she says, this should not preclude behaving with natural warmth and spontaneity. Indeed, these qualities may be needed to support patients through a stressful interview process.

Similarly, the interviewer must try to use natural, commonly understood language and avoid jargon or technical terms. The interviewer must communicate his or her intention to keep the patient as safe as possible, whatever the circumstances. Thus, while one must at times set limits on the behavior of an agitated, threatening, or abusive patient, one should never be attacking or rejecting.

Empathy is an important quality in psychiatric interviewing. While sympathy is an expression of agreement or support for another, empathy entails putting oneself in another's place and experiencing his or her state of mind. Empathy comprises both one's experiencing of another person's mental state and the expression of that understanding to the other person (Barrett-Lennard, 1981). For example, in listening to a man talk about the death of his wife, the interviewer may allow himself or herself to resonate empathetically with the patient's feelings of loneliness and desolation. Based on this resonance, he or she might respond, "After a loss like that, it feels as if the world is completely empty".

As a mode of listening, empathy is an important way of understanding the patient; as a mode of response, it is important in building rapport and alliance. Patients who feel great emotional distance from the interviewer may make empathic understanding difficult or impossible. Thus, the interviewer's inability to empathize may itself be a clue to the patient's state of mind.

Structure of the Interview

In reconnaissance phases, the interviewer inquires about broad areas of symptomatology, functioning, or life course: "Have you ever had long periods when you felt very low in mood?" "How have you been getting along at work?" "Tell me what you did between high school and when you got married". In responding to such questions, patients give the interviewer leads, which then must be pursued with more detailed questioning. Leads may include references to symptoms, difficulty in functioning, interpersonal problems, ideas, states of feeling, or stressful life events. Each such lead raises questions about the nature of the underlying problem, and the interviewer must attempt to gather enough detailed information to answer these questions. Reliance on yes or no "gate questions" to rule out areas of pathology has been shown to increase the risk of missing important information.

In general, the initial reconnaissance consists of asking how the patient comes to treatment at this particular time. This is done by asking an open-ended question such as "What brings you to see me today?" or "How did you come to be in the hospital right now?" A well-organized and cooperative patient may spontaneously provide most of the needed information, with little intervention from the interviewer. However, the patient may reveal deficits in thought process, memory, or ability to communicate, which dictate more structured and narrowly focused questioning.

The patient's emotional state and attitude may also impede a smooth flow of information. For example, if the patient shows evidence of anxiety, hostility, suspiciousness, or indifference, the interviewer must first build a working alliance before trying to collect information. This usually requires acknowledging the emotions that the patient presents, helping the patient to express his or her feelings and related thoughts, and discussing these concerns in an accepting and empathic manner (Strean, 1985). As new areas of content open up, the interviewer must continue to attend to the patient's reactions, both verbal and nonverbal, and to identify and address resistance to open communication.

Setting an appropriate level of structure is an important aspect of psychiatric interviewing. Psychiatric patients may spontaneously report a low number of symptoms, and initial diagnostic impressions may be misleading (Herran *et al.*, 2001). Over the past two decades, a variety of structured interview formats have been developed for psychiatric assessment. In these interviews, the organization, content areas, and, to varying degrees, wording of the questions are standardized; vague, overly complex, leading or biased, and judgmental questions are eliminated, as is variability in the attention given to different areas of content. The major benefits of such interviews are that they ensure complete coverage of the specified areas and greatly increase the reliability of information gathered and diagnostic judgments. In addition, formats that completely specify the wording of questions can be administered by less highly trained interviewers or even as patient self-reports.

The disadvantages of highly structured interviews are that they diminish the ability to respond flexibly to the patient and preclude exploration of any areas not specified in the format. They are therefore used to best advantage for interviews with focused goals. For example, such interviews may aim to survey certain DSM V disorders, to assess the type and degree of substance abuse, or to delineate the psychological and behavioral consequences of a traumatic event. They are less useful in a general psychiatric assessment where the scope and focus of the interview cannot be preordained.

In the usual clinical situation, while the interviewer may have a standardized general plan of approach, he or she must adapt the degree of structure to the individual patient. Open-ended, nondirective questions derive from the psychoanalytic tradition. They are most useful for eliciting and following emotionally salient themes in the patient's life story and interpersonal history. Focused, highly structured questioning derives from the medical/descriptive tradition and is most useful for delineating the scope and evolution of pathological signs and symptoms. In general, one uses the least amount of structure needed to maintain a good flow of communication and cover the necessary topic areas.

Phases of the Interview

The typical interview comprises an opening, middle, and closing phase. In the opening phase, the interviewer and patient are introduced, and the purposes and procedures of the interview are set. It is generally useful for the interviewer to begin by summarizing what he or she already knows about the patient and proceeding to the patient's own account of the situation. For example, the interviewer may say, "Dr Smith has told me that you have had several episodes of depression in the past, and now you may be going into another one", or "I understand that you were brought in by the police because you were threatening people on the street. What do you think is happening with you?" or "When we spoke on the phone you said you thought your marriage was in trouble. What has been going wrong?" Such an approach orients the patient and sets a collaborative tone.

The opening phase may also include clarification of what the patient hopes to gain from the consultation. A question such as "How were you hoping I could help you with the problem you have told me about?" invites the patient to formulate and express his or her request and avoids situations in which the patient and interviewer work at cross-purposes. The interviewer must also be explicit about his or her own goals and the extent to which they fit with the patient's expectations. This is especially important when the interests of a third party, such as an employer, a family member, or a court of law, is involved.

The middle phase of the interview consists of assessing the major issues in the case and filling in enough detail to answer the salient questions and construct a working formulation. Most of the work of determining the relative importance of biological, psychological, environmental, and sociocultural contributions to the problem is done during this phase. The patient's attitudes and transferential perceptions are also monitored during this phase so that the interviewer can recognize and address barriers to communication and collaboration.

When appropriate, formal aspects of the MSE are performed during the middle phase of the interview. While most of the MSE is accomplished simply by observing the patient, certain components such as cognitive testing and review of psychotic symptoms may not fit smoothly into the rest of the interview. These are generally best covered toward the end of the interview, after the issues of greatest importance to the patient have been discussed and rapport has been established. A brief explanation that the interviewer has a few standard questions he or she needs to cover before the end of the interview serves as a bridge and minimizes the awkwardness of asking questions that may seem incongruous or pejorative.

In general, note-taking during an assessment interview is helpful to the interviewer and not disruptive of rapport with the patient. Notes should be limited to brief recording of factual material such as dates, durations, symptom lists, important events, and past treatments, which might be difficult to keep in memory accurately. The interviewer must take care not to become so involved in taking notes as to lose touch with the patient. It is especially important to maintain a posture of attentive listening when the patient is talking about emotionally intense or meaningful issues. When done with interpersonal sensitivity, note-taking during an assessment interview may actually enhance rapport by communicating that what the patient says is important and worth remembering. This is to be distinguished from note-taking during psychotherapy sessions, which is more likely to diminish the treater's ability to listen and respond flexibly.

In the third or closing phase of the interview, the interviewer shares his or her conclusions with the patient, makes treatment recommendations and elicits reactions. In situations where the assessment runs longer than one session, the interviewer may sum up what has been covered in the interview and what needs to be done in subsequent sessions. Communications of this kind serve several purposes. They allow the patient to correct or add to the salient facts as understood by the interviewer. They contribute to the patient's feeling of having gained something from the interview. They are also the first step in initiating the treatment process because they present a provisional understanding of the problem and a plan for dealing with it. All treatment plans must be negotiated with the patient, including discussion of mutual goals, expected benefits, liabilities, limitations, and alternatives, if any. In many cases, such negotiations extend beyond the initial interview and may constitute the first phase of treatment.

Dimensions of Interviewing Techniques

To classify interviewing techniques, it is convenient to think about four major dimensions of interviewing style: degree of directiveness, degree of emotional support, degree of fact versus feeling orientation, and degree of feedback to the patient. The interviewer must seek a balance among these dimensions to best cover the needed topics, build rapport, and arrive at a plan of treatment.

Directiveness

Directiveness in the interview ensures that the necessary areas of information are covered and supplies whatever cognitive support the patient needs in discussing them. Table 4.6 lists interventions that are low, moderate, and high in directiveness.

Low-directive interventions request information in the broadest, most open-ended way and do not go beyond the material supplied by the patient. Moderately directive

Table 4.6 Degrees of Directiveness in the Interviewer

Directiveness	Intervention	Examples
Low	Open-ended questions	"What brings you to the hospital?" "Tell me about your current situation in life".
Low	Repetition	*Patient*: "Last night I suddenly started to feel so terrible I was afraid I was going to die". *Interviewer*: "You were afraid you were going to die".
Low	Restatement	*P*: "Nobody is on my side anymore – even my family is out to get me". *I*: "So it seems as if everyone has turned against you".
Low	Summarization	"To review what we have been discussing, over the last month you've been very low in mood, you felt overwhelmed even by small chores, and you no longer want to see any of your friends".
Low	Clarification	"You told me that it 'upsets' you to have to say no. It seems that when you say no to your boss your feeling is fear, but when you say no to your children you feel guilty".
Low	Nonverbal acknowledgment	"Uh-huh"; nodding of head.
Low	Attentive listening	In talking about the recent death of his wife, the patient became tearful and hesitant in speech. The interviewer remained silent, but attentive, allowing the patient time to express himself or herself.
Moderate	Broad-focus questions	"What do you notice about yourself lately that is different from usual?" "What is it about your job that you find stressful?"
Moderate	Use of examples	"Sometimes illness seems to be triggered by something that happens, like a change in finances or living situation, or losing someone who's close to you. Has anything like that been happening to you?"

(Continued)

Table 4.6 *(Cont'd)*

Directiveness	Intervention	Examples
Moderate	Confrontation	"You told me you got a 'terrible' evaluation at work, but in 9 of 10 categories, your rating was actually excellent". "You don't feel the medicine does you any good, but whenever you've stopped it, you've had to go back into the hospital. How do you account for that?"
Moderate	Interpretation	"Part of the tension between you and your wife is that you forget things she tells you. Perhaps this is what you do when you are angry at her".
High	Narrow-focus questions	"Do you have trouble getting to sleep or staying asleep?" "How much alcohol do you drink in a week?"
High	Question repetition	*I*: "How has your daily routine changed in the last month?" *P*: "I used to like to read, but now I don't anymore. My husband thinks I would feel better if I pushed myself to keep busy, but I tell him that this dizziness makes it impossible for me to do anything. I don't know what to think anymore". *I*: "How else has your routine changed lately?"
High	Redirection	*P*: "I've always thought that my father's personality caused a lot of my troubles in life". *I*: "I'd like to hear more of your thoughts about that, but first I need to get a clearer picture of what's been happening with you lately. When did you decide to make the appointment with me?"
High	Change of topics	"You mentioned before that your brother had similar problems to yours. Can you tell me how many brothers and sisters you have, and if they've had any emotional problems?" "We've been talking about your marriage, but now I'd like to know something about your work".
High	Limit-setting	"I'm going to have to interrupt you because there are a few more things we need to cover in the time left". "I know you feel restless, but I have to ask you to try to stay in your chair and concentrate on what we're talking about".

interventions are narrower in focus and may extend beyond what the patient himself or herself has said. For example, confrontation makes the patient aware of paradoxes or inconsistencies in the material and requests him or her to resolve them; interpretation requests the patient to consider explanations or connections that had not previously occurred to him or her. Highly directive interventions aim to focus and restrict the patient's content or behavior. Such interventions include yes/no or symptom–checklist-type questions and requests for the patient to modify behaviors that impede the progress of the interview.

Supportiveness

Patients vary considerably in the degree of emotional and cognitive support they need in the interview. Table 4.7 lists examples of emotionally supportive interventions. Each such intervention supports the patient's sense of security and self-esteem. While some patients may come to the interview feeling safe and confident, others have considerable anxiety about being criticized, ridiculed, rejected, taken advantage of, or attacked (literally so in the case of some psychotic patients).

Overt manifestations of insecurity range widely from fearful demeanor and tremulousness to requests for reassurance to haughty contemptuousness. The interviewer's task is to identify such anxiety when it arises and respond in a manner that conveys empathic understanding, acceptance, and positive regard.

Table 4.7 Supportive Interventions

Intervention	Examples
Encouragement	*Patient*: "I'm not sure I'm making any sense today doctor". *Interviewer*: "You're doing very well at describing the troubles you've been having".
Approval	"You did the right thing by coming in for an appointment". "You've been doing your best to keep going under very difficult circumstances".
Reassurance	"What you are telling me about may seem very strange to you, but many people have had similar experiences". "You feel like you will be sick forever, but with treatment you have a very good chance of feeling better soon".
Acknowledgment of affect	"You look very sad when you talk about your brother". "I have the impression that my question made you angry".
Empathic statements	"When your boyfriend doesn't call you, you feel completely helpless and unloved". "It seems unfair for you to get sick so many times while others remain well".
Nonverbal communication	Smiling, firm handshake, attentive body posture, gentle touch on shoulder.
Avoidance of affect-laden material	Interviewer elects to defer discussion or probing of topics that arouse intense feelings of anxiety, shame, or anger.

Obstructive interventions are those that (usually unintentionally) impede the flow of information and diminish rapport. Table 4.8 lists common examples of such interventions. Compound or vague questions are often confusing to the patient and may produce ambiguous or unclear answers. Biased or judgmental questions suggest what answer the

Table 4.8 Obstructive Interventions

Intervention	Examples
Suggestive or biased questions	"You haven't been feeling suicidal, have you?" "You've had six jobs in the last 2 years. I guess none of them held your interest".
Judgmental questions or statements	"How long have you been behaving so selfishly?" "What you've told me is typical of delusional thinking".
"Why" questions	"Why can't you sit still?" "Why do you keep choosing men who can't make a commitment to you?"
Ignoring the patient's leads	*Patient*: "I'm afraid I'm going to fall apart". *Interviewer*: "Have you had any odd experiences, such as hearing voices?" *P*: "No, but I just feel as though I can't cope and I wanted to talk to someone about it". *I*: "Has your sleep pattern or appetite changed?" *P*: "Well, I don't sleep as well as I used to, but it's getting through the days that's the hardest". *I*: "Have you had any suicidal thought?", etc.
Crowding the patient with questions	*P*: "I just can't get it out of my mind that this cancer of mine is a punishment of some kind because I …" *I*: "Have you been in a low mood or been tearful?"
Compound questions	"Have you ever heard voices or thought that other people were out to harm you?"
Vague questions	"Do you feel socially self-conscious a lot?" "How much trouble do you have with your memory?"
Minimization or dismissal	*P*: "I don't seem to be able to enjoy my life as much as I think I should". *I*: "You're doing well at your job and have a nice family – you're probably just feeling some minor stress".
Premature advice or reassurance	*P*: "I've been having terrible headaches and I forget a lot of things. There's nothing wrong with my brain, is there?" *I*: "Headaches and forgetfulness are very common and are probably due to some minor cause in your case". *P*: "I've started to have thoughts that I married the wrong man and I should leave my husband". *I*: "Maybe the two of you ought to take some time away together".
Nonverbal questions	Sitting at a distance, yawning, looking at watch, fidgeting, frowning, rolling of eyes.

interviewer wants to hear or that he or she does not approve of what the patient is saying. "Why" questions often sound critical or invite rationalizations. "How" questions better serve the purposes of the interview ("How did you come to change jobs?" rather than "Why did you change jobs?"). Other interventions are obstructive because they disregard the patient's feeling state or what he or she is trying to say. Paradoxically, this may include premature reassurance or advice, that is, when given before the interviewer has explored and understood the issue, this has the effect of cutting off feelings and coming to a premature closure.

Fact versus Feeling Orientation

Interviews differ in the degree to which they focus on factual–objective- versus feeling–meaning-oriented material. Table 4.9 and Table 4.10 provide examples of interventions of both types. The interviewer must determine what the salient issues are in a given case and develop the focus accordingly. For example, at one extreme, the principal task in assessing a cyclically occurring mood disorder might be to delineate precisely the symptoms, time course, and treatment response of the illness. At the other end of the spectrum might be a patient with a circumscribed difficulty in living, such as the inability to achieve an intimate, lasting love relationship. In such a case, the interviewer may focus not only on the facts of the patient's interactions with others but also on the feelings, fantasies, and thoughts associated with such relationships.

Table 4.9 Fact-oriented Interventions in the Psychiatric Interview

Intervention	Examples
Questions about symptoms	"Do the voices seem to come from within your own head or from outside?" "When did you first begin to check your door lock many times before going out?"
Questions about behavior	"What do you do when you fly into a rage – do you yell, hit the furniture, or hit people?" "Since you've had your pain, how is your daily routine different than it used to be?"
Questions about events	"What was the next thing you did after you took the overdose of medication?" "What led up to your decision to move out of your parents' home?"
Request for biographical data	"Who lived with you when you were growing up?" "How many times have you been in a psychiatric hospital?" "Tell me about your close relationships with women".
Requests for medical data	"What medicines do you take?" "What conditions do you see a doctor for?"

Table 4.10 Feeling-oriented Interventions in the Psychiatric Interview

Intervention	Examples
Questions about feelings in specific situations	"Some people might have been angry in the situation you told me about. Did you feel that way?" "How did you feel when your doctor told you that you had a heart attack?" "I've noticed your voice got much quieter when you answered my last question. What were you feeling just then?"
Questions or comments about emotional themes or patterns	"Growing up, you never felt like you measured up to your mother's expectations. Do you feel that same way in your marriage?"
Questions or comments about the personal meaning of events	"You are concerned about becoming enraged at your daughter. When she disregards your wishes, what do you feel that means about you as a parent?"

Feedback

Interviews differ in how much the interviewer conveys to the patient of his or her own thoughts, feelings, conclusions, and recommendations. Table 4.11 presents common types of feedback from the interviewer. Judicious statements about the interviewer's ongoing thoughts and feelings can be used to pose questions or make clarifications or interpretations while enhancing rapport and trust. Communication of factual information, formulations of the problem, and treatment recommendations are the foundations of joint treatment planning with the patient. Responding to questions and giving advice may serve an educational purpose as well as enhancing the alliance. When responding to requests for advice or information, the interviewer must first take care to be sure of what is being asked, and for what reason.

There is little systematic data on the superiority of one clinical interviewing style over another, but what there are suggest that many styles can be used effectively. Rutter and his colleagues have investigated this question in a series of naturalistic and experimental studies of interviews of parents in a child psychiatry clinic (Cox *et al.*, 1981, 1988; Rutter *et al.*, 1981). The major findings of these studies are as follows:

1. Active, structured techniques are no better than nondirective styles in eliciting positive findings (i.e., areas of pathology). However, active techniques are better in eliciting more detailed and thorough information in areas where pathology is found and are also better at delineating areas without pathology.
2. An active, fact-gathering style does not prevent the interviewer from effectively eliciting emotional reactions from informants.
3. Use of open questions, direct requests for feelings, interpretations of feelings, and expressions of sympathy are associated with greater expression of emotions by informants.

Table 4.11 Feedback in the Psychiatric Interview

Intervention	Examples
Sharing of ongoing thoughts	"As you were talking I began to wonder if you had ever lost anyone very close to you". "As I hear your story it occurs to me that you've been an outsider every place you've lived in".
Sharing of subjective reactions	"What you are saying makes me feel quite sad". "You've told me how you left treatment with your last psychiatrist, but I still feel a bit confused about what happened". "I notice I'm feeling somewhat tense right now and I wonder if you might be feeling it too".
Imparting of information	"About 75% of people with your condition respond well to medication". "The tendency to develop the kind of symptoms you have described runs in families, and probably is inherited".
Proposing a formulation	"I think the immediate cause of your depression and insomnia is your heavy drinking". "When you are under stress you tend not to think clearly and to develop unrealistic fears. It seems as though your present stress comes from the way you and your family are getting along at home".
Making treatment recommendations	"In order for you to keep safe and begin treatment I think it would be best to go into the hospital for a while". "Medication should help you get out of your depression much faster. When you are feeling better, it would be a good idea for us to try to understand how you got so isolated from your friends and family".
Advice	"It might be better not to decide about changing jobs until you're feeling back to your regular self".
Response to questions	*Patient*: "What type of psychiatrist are you, doctor?" *Interviewer*: "I'm a general psychiatrist who uses medication and psychotherapy. I also have a special interest in anxiety disorder". *P*: "Have you ever seen another patient like me?" *I*: "I can answer your question better if you tell me what there is about you that I might have never seen before". *P*: "Do you think I'm a terrible person?" *I*: "I don't think you are terrible, but I wonder what you think about yourself that you would ask me that".

4. Less activity on the interviewer's part is associated with more informant talkativeness and spontaneous emotional expression. Less directive techniques also tend to produce more emotional responses at times when they are not specifically requested. Conversely, more active styles of asking about feelings may be more effective for informants who are low in spontaneous emotional expression.
5. In summary, techniques that actively elicit both facts and emotions are likely to produce the richest, most detailed database. When skillfully used, these do not impair the doctor–patient relationship.

References

Abramowitz JS (1997) Effectiveness of psychological and pharmacological treatments for obsessive–compulsive disorder: A quantitative review. *Journal of Consulting and Clinical Psychology* 65, 44–52.

Andreasen N and Hoevk PR (1982) The predictive value of adjustment disorders. A follow-up study. *American Journal of Psychiatry* 134, 584–590.

Banmohl J and Jaffe JH (1995) History of alcohol and drug abuse treatment in the United States, in *Encyclopedia of Drugs and Alcohol*, Vol. 3 (ed. Jaffe JM). Macmillan, New York.

Barlow DH (1988) *Anxiety and Its Disorders – The Nature and Treatment of Anxiety and Panic*. Guilford Press, New York.

Barlow DM, Gorman JM, Shear MK *et al.* (2000) Cognitive–behavioral therapy, imipramine, or their combination for panic disorder: A randomized controlled trial. *Journal of American Medical Association* 283, 2529–2536.

Barrett-Lennard GT (1981) The empathy cycle. Refinement of a nuclear concept. *Journal of Counseling Psychology* 28, 91–100.

Bateman A and Fonagy P (2001) Treatment of borderline personality disorder with psychoanalytically oriented partial hospitalization: An 18-month follow-up. *American Journal of Psychiatry* 158, 36–42.

Baxter LR (1992) Neuroimaging studies of obsessive–compulsive disorder. *Psychiatric Clinics of North America* 15(1), 841–884.

Bellack AS and Mueser KT (1993) Psychosocial treatment of schizophrenia. *Schizophrenia Bulletin* 19, 317–336.

Blazer DC, Hughes D and George LK (1991) Generalized anxiety disorder, in *Psychiatric Disorders in America. The Epidemiologic Catchment Area Study* (ed. Robins LN). Free Press, New York, pp. 180–203.

Brenner JD and Marmer CR (1998) *Trauma, Memory and Dissociation*. American Psychiatric Press, Washington, DC.

Carpenter W and Buchanan RW (1994) Schizophrenia. *New England Journal of Medicine* 330, 681–690.

Clarkin JF, Levy KN, Lezenweger MF, *et al.* (2007). Evaluating three treatments for borderline personality disorder: A multiwave study. *American Journal of Psychiatry* 164(6), 922–928.

Cloninger CR (1987) A systematic model for clinical description and classification of personality variants. *Archives of General Psychiatry* 44, 573–588.

Cloninger R, Martin RL, Guze SB *et al.* (1986) A prospective follow-up and family study of somatization in men and women. *American Journal of Psychiatry* 143, 873–878.

Cloninger CR, Surakic DM and Przybeck TR (1993) A psychobiological model of temperament and character. *Archives of General Psychiatry* 50, 975–990.

Coccaro ER and Kavoussi RJ (1997) Fluoxetine and impulsive-aggressive behavior in personality-disordered subjects. *Archives of General Psychiatry* 45, 1081–1088.

Cox A, Holbrook D and Rutter M (1981) Psychiatric interviewing techniques VI. Experimental study. Eliciting feelings. *British Journal of Psychiatry* 139, 144–152.

Cox A, Rutter M and Holbrook D (1988) Psychiatric interviewing techniques. A second experimental study: Eliciting feelings. *British Journal of Psychiatry* 152, 64–72.

Davis JM (1975) Overview: Maintenance therapy in psychiatry. I. Schizophrenia. *American Journal of Psychiatry* 132, 1237–1245.

Elkin I, Shea T, Watkins J *et al.* (1989) National Institute of Mental Health Treatment of Depression Collaborative Research Program. General effectiveness of treatments. *Archives of General Psychiatry* 46, 971–982.

Ford CV (1995) Dimensions of somatization and hypochondriasis. *Neurologic Clinics* 13, 241–253.

Ford CV and Foulks DG (1985) Conversion disorders. An overview. *Psychosomatics* 26, 371–374.

Fyer AJ, Munnuzza S, Gallops MS *et al.* (1990) Familial transmission of simple phobias and fears: A preliminary report. *Archives of General Psychiatry* 47, 252–256.

Goddard AW and Charney DS (1997) Toward an integrated neurolobiology of panic disorder. *Journal of Clinical Psychiatry* 58(Suppl.), 4–11.

Goodwin FK and Jamison KR (1990) *Manic–Depressive Illness*. Oxford University Press, New York.

Greenberg WM, Rosenfeld D and Ortege E (1995) Adjustment disorder: An admission diagnosis. *American Journal Psychiatry* 152, 459–461.

Halmi K (ed.) (1992) *The Psychobiology and Treatment of Anorexia Nervosa and Bulimia Nervosa*. American Psychiatric Press, Washington, DC.

Heim C, Ehlert U and Helhammer DH (2000) The potential role of hypocortisolism in pathophysiology of stress related bodily disorders. *Psychoneuroendocrinology* 25, 1–35.

Herran A, Sierra-Biddle D, deSantiago A *et al.* (2001) Diagnostic accuracy in the first 5 minutes of a psychiatric interview. *Psychotherapy and Psychosomatics* 70, 141–144.

Insel TR (1992) Toward a neuroanatomy of obsessive–compulsive disorder. *Archives of General Psychiatry* 49, 739–744.

Janowsky DS, El-Yousef MK and Davis JM (1974) Playing the name game. Interpersonal maneuvers of manic patients. *American Journal of Psychiatry* 131, 250–255.

Johnson C and Connors ME (1987) *The Etiology and Treatment of Bulimia Nervosa*. Basic Books, New York.

Jorgensen P, Bennedson B, Christensen J *et al.* (1996) Acute and transient psychotic disorder. Comorbidity with personality disorder. *Acta Psychiatrica Scandinavica* 94(6), 460–464.

Katz L, Fleisher W, Kjernisted K *et al.* (1996) A review of the psychobiology and pharmacotherapy of posttraumatic stress disorder. *Canadian Journal of Psychiatry* 41, 233–238.

Keck PE, McElroy SL and Strakowski SM (1996) New developments in the pharmacological treatments of schizoaffective disorder. *Journal of Clinical Psychiatry* 57, 41–48.
Kellner R (1987) Hypochondriasis and somatization. *Journal of American Medical Association* 258, 2718–2722.
Kendler KS (1991) Mood-incongruent psychotic affective illness. A historical empirical review. *Archives of General Psychiatry* 48, 362–369.
Kendler KS, Masterson CL, Ungaro R *et al.* (1984) A family history study of schizophrenia-related personality disorders. *American Journal of Psychiatry* 143, 424–427.
Kluft RP and Fine CG (1993) *Clinical Perspectives on Multiple Personality Disorder.* Psychiatric Press, Washington, DC.
Kotrla KJ and Weinberger DR (1995) Brain imaging in schizophrenia. *Annual Review of Medicine* 46, 113–122.
Lazare A (1981) Current concepts in psychiatry. Conversion symptoms. *New England Journal of Medicine* 305, 745–748.
Leigh H and Reiser M (1992) (eds) Confusion, delerium, and dementia. Organic brain syndromes and the elderly patient, in *The Patient: Biological, Psychological, and Social Dimensions of Medical Practice*, 3rd edn. Plenum Press, New York.
Lipowski ZJ (1984) Organic mental disorders – An American perspective. *British Journal of Psychiatry* 144, 542–546.
Lishman WA (1978) *Organic Psychiatry*. Blackwell, Oxford.
LoPiccolo J (1985) Diagnosis and treatment of male sexual dysfunction. *Journal of Sex & Marital Therapy* 2, 215–232.
Maber BA (1992) Delusions. Contemporary etiological hypotheses. *Psychiatric Annals* 22, 260–264.
Manschreck TC (1996) Delusional disorder. The recognition and management of paranoia. *Journal of Clinical Psychiatry* 57(Suppl.), 32–38.
Marks IM (1987) *Fears, Phobias and Rituals: Panic, Anxiety and Their Disorders*. Oxford University Press, New York.
Marks I, Lovell K, Noshirvani H *et al.* (1998) Treatment of post-traumatic stress disorder by exposure and/or cognitive restructuring: A controlled study. *Archives of General Psychiatry* 55, 317–325.
Marshall WL and Barbaree HE (1990) An integrated theory of the etiology of sexual offending, in *Handbook of Sexual Assault. Issues, Theories, and Treatment of the Offender* (eds Marshall WL, Laws DN and Barbaree HE). Plenum Press, New York, pp. 257–275.
Merlett GA (1998) Addictive behaviors, etiology and treatment. *Annual Review of Psychology* 39, 223–252.
Millon T (1996) *Disorders of Personality: DSM-IV and Beyond*. John Wiley & Sons, Inc., New York.
Milrod B, Busch F, Leon AC *et al.* (2000) Open trial of psychodynamic therapy for panic disorder: A pilot study. *American Journal of Psychiatry* 157, 1878–1880.
Min SK and Lee BO (1997) Laterality in somatization. *Psychosomatic Medicine* 59, 236–240.
Nemiah J (1961) Psychological conflict, in *Foundations of Psychopathology* (ed. Nemiah H). Oxford University Press, New York, pp. 35–55.

Nesse RM and Berridge KC (1997) Psychoactive drug use in evolutionary perspective. *Science* 278, 63–66.

Nurnberg HG, Raskin M, Levine PE *et al.* (1991) Hierarchy of DSM-III R. Criteria efficiency for the diagnosis of borderline personality disorder. *Journal of Personality Disorders* 5, 211–244.

Popkin MK (1994) Syndromes of brain dysfunction presenting with cognitive impairment or behavioral disturbance. Delirium, dementia, and mental disorders due to a general medical condition, in *The Medical Basis of Psychiatry*, 2nd edn (eds Winokur G and Clayton PJ). WB Saunders, Philadelphia, pp. 17–37.

Prescott CA and Kendler KS (1999) Genetic and environmental contributions to alcohol abuse and dependence in a population-based sample of male twins. *American Journal of Psychiatry* 156, 34–40.

Rutter M, Cox A, Egert S *et al.* (1981) Psychiatric interviewing techniques IV. Experimental study. Four contrasting styles. *British Journal of Psychiatry* 138, 456–465.

Sensky T, Turkington D, Kingdon D *et al.* (2000) A randomized controlled trail of cognitive–behavioral therapy for persistent symptoms in schizophrenia resistant to medication. *Archives of General Psychiatry* 57, 165–272.

Siever LJ and Davis KL (1985) Overview: Toward a dysregulation hypothesis of depression. *American Journal of Psychiatry* 142, 1017–1033.

Siever LJ, Bernstein DP and Silverman JM (1991) Schizotypal, paranoid, and schizoid personality disorders: A review of their current status. *Journal of Personality Disorders* 5, 178–193.

Strean H (1985) *Resolving Resistances in Psychotherapy*. John Wiley & Sons, Inc., New York.

Susser E, Fennig S, Jandorf L *et al.* (1995) Epidemiology, diagnosis and course of brief psychoses. *American Journal of Psychiatry* 152, 1745–1748.

Svartberg M, Stile TC, Seltzer MH (2004) Randomized, controlled trial of the effectiveness of short-term dynamic psychotherapy and cognitive therapy for cluster C personality disorders. *American Journal of Psychiatry* 161, 810–817.

Tarnepolsky A and Berlowitz M (1987) Borderline personality – A review of recent research. *British Journal of Psychiatry* 151, 724–734.

Thase M and Howland RH (1995) Biological processes in depression. An updated review and integration, in *Handbook of Depression* (eds Beckham E and Leber W). Guilford Press, New York.

Tsuang M and Faraone S (1990) *The Genetics of Mood Disorders*. Johns Hopkins University Press, Baltimore.

Winokur G, Monahan P, Coryell W *et al.* (1996) Schizophrenia and affective disorder – Distinct entities or a continuum? An analysis based on a 6-year follow-up. *Comprehensive Psychiatry* 37, 77–87.

Zuckerman M (1996) The psychobiological model for impulsive unsocialized sensation seeking. A comparative approach. *Neuropsychobiology* 34, 125–129.

CHAPTER

5 Psychiatric Interviews: Special Populations

Randon Welton and Jerald Kay

There is a popular image of the psychiatric interview where the patient and clinician sit comfortably in soft leather chairs in the psychiatrist's office surrounded by objets d'art and built-in bookshelves. The patient speaks clearly, honestly, and succinctly about his or her problem. The psychiatrist listens intently and understands thoroughly what is being said. This mutual understanding allows the therapy to begin effectively and proceed quickly to its successful conclusion. All too often, the reality of psychiatric practice reflects more challenging situations.

In this chapter, we shall be examining a number of special, but nonetheless common, clinical circumstances and patient populations that tend to bend the frame of the traditional psychiatric interview. There are an infinite number of special circumstances of course, and this chapter could hardly list, much less discuss, them all. Instead we will be looking at examples within two major themes. Sometimes the interview is extraordinary because of the circumstances surrounding the interview. At other times, psychiatrists will be interacting with a distinct population of patients; patients that inherently require an alteration of our approach. These situations require extra thoughtfulness and adaptation on the part of the clinician.

Included under the heading of *Special Circumstances* are patients located on *Inpatient Units*, on *Medical Wards*, or in the *Emergency Department* (ED). The acuity of these patients and the lack of privacy in these locations contribute to the difficulty of the interview. Another set of special circumstances occurs in *Mass Casualty or Disaster* scenarios. In those calamities, the psychiatrist may be responsible to assess large numbers of patients in orthodox settings.

Even when the interview takes place in a more traditional setting, there are *Special Populations* that may challenge the psychiatrist. These include patients with severe *Psychotic Symptoms* or significant *Suicidality*. Interviewing *Children and Adolescents* can pose a challenge for the non-subspecialist. Also included in these special populations are those where there is a difference in language between the patient and the psychiatrist. This creates the need to incorporate *Interpreters* into the psychiatric interview. *Cultural*

The Psychiatric Interview: Evaluation and Diagnosis, First Edition. Allan Tasman, Jerald Kay and Robert J. Ursano.

Barriers are invariably present with patients from different ethnic and racial backgrounds even when they are fluent in English. These differences add difficulty to the psychiatric interview. In these days of increasing demands and falling recruitment within psychiatry, *Telepsychiatry* is becoming an increasingly common solution to providing access to psychiatry. This new technology, however, often is accompanied by some unique issues that, if not addressed, add complexity to the clinical interview.

Psychiatric Interview in Special Circumstances

Special Circumstances – Inpatient Units

Interviewing hospitalized psychiatric patients is a routine responsibility that may lead to an insensitivity to the uniqueness of this environment. Because of the ubiquitous legal and financial demands inherent in inpatient treatment, modifications to interview style are necessary. Since a thorough history and physical examination must be documented within the first 24 hours of admission, this first encounter is likely to be the longest one-on-one interaction between the patient and psychiatrist.

This documentation of the history and physical examination must meet the standard required by regulatory agencies such as the Joint Commission for the Accreditation of Hospitals and includes, but is not limited to, assessments of the patient's preferred method of learning, patient strengths, risk to self, comprehensive psychiatric and medical history, and risk to others. Diagnoses and treatment plans are required as well. In addition, the psychiatrist will need enough information to satisfy utilization management and third-party standards for hospitalization. The time pressure to get the necessary information as quickly as possible shapes the psychiatrist's interview. In the rush to obtain the requisite information, clinicians often resort to simplified information-gathering tools such as checklists and "Yes/No" questions, which must be carefully balanced with the development of a doctor–patient relationship based on empathy and understanding.

Many inpatient units have adopted a team interview model where the psychiatrist is the collator of information rather than the collector of that information. These units see it as more cost-effective for nonphysicians to gather much of the background information. So rather than asking traditional open-ended questions about the patient's past experiences, the psychiatrist simply "signs off" on the history obtained by other mental health-care providers. This may limit the engagement in the therapeutic relationship between the patient and the psychiatrist.

The accuracy of a traditional psychiatric inpatient interview has been questioned. Researchers looked for inter-rater reliability among providers assessing 56 patients using three different methods. The methods included a traditional, unstructured diagnostic assessment (TDA), the Structured Clinical Interview for the DSM – Clinical version (SCID), and a Computer-Assisted Diagnostic Interview (CADI), which utilized questions based on DSM-IV algorithms. Following the individual interviews, the interviewers met to come up with a consensus diagnosis. Compared to the consensus diagnosis, the unstructured TDA was in agreement 53.8% of the time, considerably less than the structured approaches (SCID – 85.7%, CADI – 85.7%) (Miller *et al.*, 2001). The same facility then looked at agreement between the diagnosis in the ED and the ultimate diagnosis on the inpatient unit. It used the same CADI to evaluate 39 patients in the ED and then reevaluated them on the inpatient unit with another provider using the CADI. This was compared to two groups who received TDAs in both the ED and the inpatient unit. The two TDA arms combined had 66 patients. Looking at inter-rater reliability found "poor" to "fair" agreement (45.5–54.5%) with the TDA, while using the CADI resulted in "excellent" agreement (79.5%) (Miller, 2001).

A final study by this group looked at the impact the assessment had on patient care. The use of the CADI ensured that the interview would cover all of the key criteria necessary to screen for the major DSM-IV criteria. Because it was preloaded with the DSM-IV algorithms, it would also cover all of the criteria when there had been a positive screening. The interviewer using a traditional diagnostic assessment on average asked only half of the key criteria screening questions and asked slightly less than half of the DSM criteria for the likely diagnoses. In these patients, who had been randomly assigned to the interviews based on their arrival at the hospital, the length of stay for those receiving the CADI was an average of 4.8 days less than those receiving the TDA (Miller, 2002). These studies did not address differences in long-term outcome nor the patients' experiences in the various approaches.

The challenge for the inpatient psychiatrist then is to obtain the diagnostic accuracy of a structured or algorithmic interview while preserving the open-ended questions and empathic connection of the traditional approaches. Working on an inpatient unit requires the psychiatrist to perform a difficult balancing act. The pace, external accountability requirements, and diagnostic precision required for the inpatient admission will challenge a slower-paced traditional interview. Often relying on information provided by others and the use of more structured and less engaging interviewing techniques is attractive. The cost of this accommodation may be a decrease in the quality and significance of the relationships between the inpatient provider and his or her patients. Although no simple solution exists to this tension, the inpatient psychiatrist can utilize a few techniques to balance these positions:

- When possible, interview the patient after the other providers have collected their information. The psychiatrist can then refer to the information that others have obtained and ask the patient to expand on it. This demonstrates that the psychiatrist has some basic understanding of the patient but wants additional information.
  - *Example* – The previous interviewer recorded: Academic history – "Graduated High School in 13 years; a few classes at community college". The psychiatrist asks: "I see that you needed an additional year to graduate high school and then went to college for a while. Tell me about that".
- Continue to ask open-ended questions, especially at the beginning of the interview. Ignoring the patient's perspective on why he or she was brought into the hospital can damage the development of a therapeutic alliance and limit the clinician's understanding.
- Continue to make empathic statements rather than exclusively elicit symptoms.
  - *Example* – The patient has a chronic history of highly critical auditory hallucinations. "I see that you have heard voices for a long time and they say some pretty bad things about you. That must be horrible. How have you managed to deal with that for all of these years?"
- Aid in the development of a positive "institutional transference" by helping the patient build trust in the entire team and not just the psychiatrist. Utilizing and praising the

work done by the other team members can aid in this. Stress the ongoing communication among the team about the patient's particular situation and treatment plan. If possible, have them interact with multiple team members at a time along with the psychiatrist.

Summary of Recommendations

- Structured evaluations may be helpful.
- Do not neglect displays of empathy and opportunities to build rapport.
- Ask open-ended questions whenever possible.
- Purposefully develop a therapeutic alliance among the patient, the psychiatrist, and the rest of the team.

Special Circumstance – Medical Wards

Although the consulting psychiatrist first and foremost has the patient's best interest at heart, the principle reason for the consultation, nevertheless, is to assist the medical or surgical provider who initiated the consult. Depending on the culture of the hospital, these providers may be asking for the psychiatrist to take over the management of the patient's psychiatric issues while on the medical ward. In other facilities, the consulting psychiatrist is merely asked for advice on how to manage the patient and does not take an active treatment role.

The patient must understand the role of the consulting psychiatrist and that information obtained by the psychiatrist during an interview may be conveyed to the treating team. If this is not clarified from the outset, the psychiatrist can be placed in an awkward position of either knowing key elements of the patient's history that he or she does not relate to the treatment team request or of betraying the patient's confidence. There are often concerns about privacy. Although some patients will have single rooms and can be assessed in privacy, the consult on the medical ward often takes place in a room that is shared with at least one other patient. The patient's medical condition may make it impossible to move the consultation to a more private setting. These factors necessitate significant changes in the initial interview. Both the patient and psychiatrist must acknowledge and accept the lack of privacy and confidentiality as well as the dual agency of the consulting psychiatrist.

The medically ill patient presents some other significant challenges. These include gathering and understanding comprehensive details of the medical or surgical condition that necessitated hospitalization. The consultant psychiatrist often returns to reading textbooks or review articles. Drug–drug interactions in these patients may also be daunting. The psychiatrist must appreciate the psychiatric manifestations of unfamiliar medications and their interactions. Again, there must be a willingness to research these issues.

As part of the consult, the psychiatrist must routinely address behavioral medicine issues in addition to elucidating specific psychiatric diagnoses. Assessing the patient's psychosocial adjustment and how it impacts on the patient's health and response to treatment falls squarely into the consulting psychiatrist's purview.

- *Example* – A 55-year-old man was admitted to a medical ward on numerous occasions for uncontrolled hypertension. While on the unit his blood pressure was well controlled with medications, within days of discharge his blood pressure rose dangerously. When asked, he insisted that he was taking his medication as prescribed and was following the other behavioral suggestions of the treatment regimen. The frustrated treatment team had asked for a consult to evaluate for malingering or factitious illness. The psychiatrist took an empathic, nonjudgmental approach with the patient, openly assuming that the patient was doing what he could to keep himself healthy. As the patient became more comfortable with the psychiatrist, this proud man disclosed that he did not have the financial resources to take his medication as prescribed and was in fact only able to afford to take the prescription "every three or four days". The psychiatrist could then assume a liaison role to the team to help them negotiate the financial aspects of his care.

The lack of comfort with managing psychiatric illnesses on the medical ward goes both ways. Often the treatment team will be uncomfortable with the patient's mental illness and have only a vague idea of what he or she would like the psychiatrist to do for him or her. This lack of clarity can be confusing for the patient and treatment team as well as for the psychiatrist. The treatment team may even consult mental health without informing the patients that they are doing so. When the psychiatrist shows up in the room, these patients can be surprised and sometimes offended that their providers have consulted mental health care without their knowledge.

There are some basic steps that the psychiatrist can take to improve the quality and value of the interview on a medical or surgical ward.

- *Specify the question to be answered* – As a consultant, the psychiatrist assists the medical team. The treatment team must, therefore, play a role in defining the focus of the psychiatrist's interview. No matter how brilliant the information obtained and relayed by the psychiatrist is, if it does not answer the team's question, then the consultation is not successful. Often the team does not fully understand what they want and will send a consult request that says in essence "See this patient". In those situations, the consultant should talk first with the team to clarify what information would be the most helpful. Are they looking for help with diagnosis? Are they concerned about the patient's current or proposed medication regimen? Do they have questions about the patient's capacity to make informed decisions? Some authors have referred to this as the "center of gravity" for the consult. The psychiatrist assists the patient by helping the medical team understand what questions they have about the patient (Philbrick *et al.*, 2012). Frequently, the initial psychiatric consult may be inappropriate or impossible.
  - *Example* – "35-year-old recently diagnosed with cancer. Patient is crying. Please evaluate".
  - *Example* – "54-year-old chronic alcoholic. He has failed numerous rehabs. He needs to stop drinking. Please assess and treat".

  One of the most important aspects of the consultation is helping the medical team understand and accept the limits of what psychiatric consultation can provide them and their patient (Nichita and Buckley, 2007; Perry and Viederman, 1981a).
- *Dealing with Skeptical Staff Members* – Unfortunately, the psychiatrist must occasionally deal with medical and surgical staff that neither understand the impact and importance of mental illness nor value the input of the psychiatrist. Often a psychiatry consult appears to team members as the most expedient way to relieve

themselves of a difficult patient. Explaining the limitations and value of a psychiatric interview and consultation can again be extremely helpful for the patient and the consulting team. The psychiatrist does not want to remove a patient's sadness over tragic events (e.g., the diagnosis of metastatic cancer). A brief consultation will not change chronic behavioral problems and cannot take the place of ongoing outpatient therapy. The consultant can, however, point the team in the right direction while recognizing that the bulk of the work must be completed elsewhere.

- *Lack of Confidentiality* – As the consulting team is the primary recipient of information, the psychiatrist must explain the limits of confidentiality to the patient at the beginning of the interview. The psychiatrist is there to help the medical team provide care. The information obtained may be conveyed to the team if it is important in the patient's medical care. The consult will be included in the general medical record and can be accessed by a host of personnel (Wise and Rundell, 2005). Of course, the consulting psychiatrist still has some discretion. Issues that might unduly embarrass the patient and will not directly impact patient care can usually be expressed in a tactful fashion.
  - *Example* – A 45-year-old female with metastatic breast cancer is being seen for depression. She discloses that her marriage recently ended when her husband announced that he was homosexual and left her for another man. The psychiatrist records: "Discussed the painful ending of her marriage".
- *Lack of Privacy* – When the interview takes place in a multi-bed room, the psychiatrist may pull the curtain shut for the illusion of privacy but his or her voice will easily carry to the other beds. If no private interview room is available or feasible, the patient can be positioned so that he or she is turned away from his or her roommate. The psychiatrist should speak softly but must ensure that the patient can hear and understand him or her. The lack of privacy should not prevent the psychiatrist from broaching potentially uncomfortable topics such as substance abuse and suicidality. Euphemisms and generalities can be used to start the conversation, but at some point the clinician will need to ask about them directly.
- *Distractions* – Although there is no way to prevent other medical personnel from interrupting the interview, nursing staff can be asked if there is anything they need from the patient before starting the interview. This should help minimize distractions. Politely insist that the television and other entertainment be turned off during the course of the interview.
- *Visitors* – Since some wards have restricted visiting hours and some visitors come from long distances, it often seems uncaring to simply ask them to leave. Working around the visitor's schedule is a kind and compassionate thing to do if possible. Those gestures can help create an instant therapeutic rapport with the patient. If, however, the psychiatrist lacks such flexibility, he or she can apologize to the patient and visitors and explain the need to interview the patient in private. Direct them to a nearby waiting room and be sure to notify them when the interview is finished.
- *Monitor Your Attitude* – Because the medical/surgical ward is often unfamiliar and uncomfortable to the psychiatrist, he or she can unconsciously adopt attitudes that are not therapeutic. Being surrounded by a "medical" environment, the psychiatrist might tend to function with a strictly biological focus. The psychiatrist adopting this unempathic stance directs his or her attention only to pertinent positive and negative

signs and symptoms, gathering much of the information from the medical records and staff members. This psychiatrist may stand by the bedside, simply confirming information already obtained from the record and adopt an attitude of the detached, benevolent authority. His or her recommendations would focus solely on laboratory studies and medication changes, ignoring psychological or social interventions. On the other hand, the psychiatrist, surrounded by poorly understood medical terminology, can overly identify with the patient. He or she can become enraged by perceived slights the patient has received from the staff and criticize the direction and pace of treatment even when he or she does not have a good understanding of the medical issues. The goal of the psychiatrist is to maintain a middle ground where he or she is more medically focused and interactive than in a traditional interview but still takes the time to let the patient explain his or her views (Perry and Viederman, 1981b).

- *Mental Status* – A significant number of psychiatry consultations center on the cognitive functioning of the patient. Up to 25% of consultations may be for some form of competency or capacity evaluation (Wise and Rundell, 2005). In addition, the psychiatrist is often asked to evaluate for confusion and/or delirium. Although the assessment of a patient's mental status may not always require the formal administration of a mental status examination, in these particular situations, the formal cognitive exam plays a pivotal role. Moreover, cognitive impairment may go undetected by nonpsychiatric medical personnel as well as by psychiatrists if there is not a deliberate exploration of those issues. The patient's social skills and polite conversation can compensate for cognitive impairment unless attention, concentration, memory, and executive functioning are specifically addressed. In order to assess cognitive functioning in a systematic way, it is advised that the psychiatrist utilize a standardized instrument such as the Folstein Mini-Mental Status Examination or the Montreal Cognitive Assessment (Wise and Rundell, 2005).
- *Collateral Information* – Especially when there is a component of cognitive impairment, patients may not be the best source of information about their current and recent life experiences and mental functioning. Even the most impaired patient deserves the psychiatrist's best effort at establishing rapport and utilizing the patient as the "expert on themselves", but the consultant must be prepared to contact family members or friends at times to clarify the patient's situation (Wise and Rundell, 2005). Although Health Information Portability and Accountability Act concerns are not raised when a sole psychiatrist gathers information, it is always best to gain the patient's consent before contacting outsiders. During these conversations with collateral sources, the psychiatrist needs to be aware that the thrust of questions may inadvertently convey personal health information to the other person. It is best therefore to stick to general questions: "What changes have you noticed in the patient?" "What other medical or mental health issues does he or she have?" "What medications does he or she take regularly" Once the informant has brought up more focused problems such as depression, confusion, or hallucination, the psychiatrist should pursue those directly.
- *The Surprised Patient* – The psychiatrist should not be surprised that some patients will be unaware that the medical team has consulted mental health. This surprised patient can become resistant to the clinician. Hostility toward the consultant can arise through the misconception that the psychiatrist believes that the patient's problems are "all in his or

her head". For this reason, many psychiatrists insist that the team's consultation request be explained to the patient before the first visit. The psychiatrist can sometimes assuage the patient's hostility by emphasizing that understanding and addressing the psychosocial aspects of illness is an important aspect of the patient's overall medical care.

  - *Example* – A 43-year-old female has been admitted for unexplained abdominal pain. The extensive workup has been negative. The consult request reads simply "43 y/o with abdominal pain without medical cause. Evaluate and treat". She is upset with her team's giving up on her and "calling in the shrink". "That's what they do when they can't find a cause. Rather than admit they are not that smart, they blame the patient". The psychiatrist explains that he or she has been invited to provide help to the team beyond the extensive workup that has been done. "Obviously your team believes you have pain or they would not have done those tests. Sometimes, though, the stress of chronic unexplained pain or persisting illness might make the person sicker than they were before. I'm wondering if you have noticed that your pain fluctuates with stress. Is it worse when things are going poorly and better when things go well?"

- *Complicated Medical/Surgical or Medication Issues* – Do not be afraid to acknowledge your ignorance. The psychiatrist can admit to the consulting team or even the patient that additional research must be conducted to better appreciate the clinical presentation. In addition to being honest, this interaction has other advantages. It models an active style of learning to the patient that he or she can use. Asking the consulting team for an explanation of the medical issues also sets a precedent for the psychiatrist explaining some of the behavioral health or mental health aspects of the case later on. Encouraging this type of interdisciplinary communication is an important aspect of the liaison function.

Summary of Recommendations

- Clarify the question.
- Clarify the roles and responsibilities.
- Engage with the consulting team.
- Address behavioral medicine issues.
- Strive for a private, uninterrupted interview.
- Complete the mental status examination.
- Maintain an empathic relationship.

Special Circumstance – Emergency Department

Interviewing patients in the ED combines many of the difficulties found on the inpatient unit and the medical ward. A significant number of patients presenting to the ED arrive with complex and severe psychiatric issues such as psychosis, suicidality, dangerousness to others, and/or aggressive behaviors. These issues are often compounded by medical illnesses and the misuse of psychoactive substances. The psychiatrist may be called to interview patients who are intoxicated or delirious. Many of these patients will be uninterested in receiving help and can be openly confrontational. There are also patients who present to the ED for what has been termed social reasons. They are homeless and know that reporting severe psychiatric symptoms is a path to shelter and meals.

The setting of the ED interview complicates a patient evaluation. The ED often lacks private, calming locations for the interview. The patient may be separated from other patients by only a sheet that does not reach the floor. Without accompanying records, the psychiatrist has nothing more than laboratory data, the physical examination, and his or her psychiatric interview on which to base his or her assessment. The evaluation may be further complicated by the ED's attitudes toward many psychiatric patients, especially when they are repeat visitors or so-called frequent flyers. These individuals are very familiar to the ED staff, and often "getting the patient up to the ward" is their sole priority.

As in the case of the Consult-Liaison psychiatry, an important aspect of treating this patient is determining the concerns of the ED staff. Often these concerns involve issues of dangerousness or the need for hospitalization. It is important that the psychiatrist knows not only what questions the ED staff have but also what prompted those concerns.

The psychiatrist should always look for past medical records. In addition to providing past diagnoses, these can also describe previous medication trials and offer a baseline of behavior and symptoms. If no such records are available, then the psychiatrist may need further discussion with ED staff members who likely have been observing the patient's affect, thinking, and behavior for several hours. Another potentially valuable and often overlooked resource are laboratory studies. The psychiatrist will want to know which have been ordered and which results have returned. Laboratory results may point to non-psychiatric issues that need to be addressed or provide reasons to delay the interview. For example, when patients are intoxicated, the psychiatrist will want to wait until the blood alcohol levels approach legal limits as information obtained while the patient is intoxicated is suspect at best.

Once again, the complexity of the situation, the acuity of the patient, and the inevitable time crunch will test the psychiatrist's ability to utilize an unstructured interview with open-ended questions. A more directed examination of the most pressing symptoms, pertinent risk factors, and criteria for admission may be indicated. Nevertheless, the patient's past psychiatric history, social history, substance use, and recent stresses must be elucidated. When suicide is a concern, in-depth exploration and documentation of current thoughts of death and suicide, recent violent or self-destructive behavior, a past history of violence or suicide attempts, current support systems, and substance abuse must be obtained (Feinstein and Plutchik, 1990).

Reliance on checklists of psychiatric symptoms is to be avoided since this practice does not permit the patient the freedom to tell his or her story in his or her own words and to express his or her understanding of his or her current predicament. While the interview will predominately focus on the presenting problem and acute issues, the psychiatrist should try to not immediately plunge into the heart of the crisis at the outset of the interview. A few questions about the patient's background and life circumstances demonstrate a thorough interest in the patient. This can also provide valuable insight into the patient's functional level as well as sources of social support.

In the rush to gather the information required for admission or medical/legal purposes, an opportunity for crisis intervention should not be squandered. Patients are exquisitely sensitive to perceived criticism and rejection by the ED staff, and a psychiatrist who is willing to make a concerted effort and take the time necessary to understand the situation can obtain valuable insights into the patient and can provide much needed support for the patient. The psychiatrist in the ED will want to deliberately and rapidly develop a therapeutic alliance. An appreciation for the patient's past efforts at solving problems reassures the patient and helps to establish this rapport.

- Example – An unemployed 52-year-old man is brought into the Emergency Department by family concerned for his safety. He recounts numerous attempts to find work and his profound sense that he is failing his family. Being brought into the Emergency Department is humiliating proof of his failure. "Not only am I not helping them, but now they are having to watch over me like I am a child." The psychiatrist praises his devotion to his family and his persistent efforts to find work. "Many people would have quit a long time ago, but I am getting the sense that quitting is not in your personality." The psychiatrist then proposes that the patient work "just as diligently" with an outpatient therapist to get control of this depression. "The first, best step to get you back on your feet is to get this depression under control."

Supporting patients and minimizing their distress while they are in the ED is not only practicing good medicine but can also facilitate the interview process. This could be something as simple as arranging for them to receive a blanket, glass of water, or medication to decrease acute anxiety. An attitude of reasonable optimism about the efficacy of medications and psychotherapy can help set the stage for future providers. All of these can elevate the ED experience from one where the psychiatrist is simply the gatekeeper to the inpatient wards to a critical therapeutic experience for the patient (Rosenberg, 1994).

Because interviewing patients in the ED is significantly different from what most psychiatrists do day to day, there are some steps that can increase the clinician's comfort during the interview and ultimately result in the provision of better care.

- Feel safe and secure.
    - If patients represent an imminent risk to themselves or others, arrange for support that is close at hand during the interview.
        - If the patient is acutely agitated, maintain a reasonable distance so that you are out of arm's reach, yet without being so distant as to make conversation difficult.
    - *Maximize Privacy* – Some EDs will have relatively quiet rooms that can be used for more difficult or sensitive interviews such as in the case of rape. If it is safe, ask for one of these rooms to increase the patient's sense of privacy and decrease distractions and interruptions.
    - *Speak to the Patient Alone* – The patient may have friends or family members with him or her. If the patient can speak for himself or herself, visitors should leave during the interview. This will decrease their opportunities to speak for the patient, and may help the patient speak more freely and accurately.
    - After the interview is complete, family or friends can be brought into the room or can be spoken to separately to confirm details of the patient's account or to gain outside perspectives. Unless the patient has expressly given permission, the psychiatrist should not provide information about the patient's condition.
    - Even with agitated and disorganized patients, it is worthwhile to start with open-ended questions. These will help the patient feel that he or she has been heard and understood. It also allows the psychiatrist to observe the patient's mental functioning in a naturalistic setting (MacKinnon *et al.*, 2006; Meyers and Stein, 2000).

Summary of Recommendations

- Clarify the question.
- Engage with the ED staff.
- Strive for a private, uninterrupted interview.
- Ask open-ended questions whenever possible.
- Build rapport.
- Maintain an empathic relationship.

Special Circumstance – Mass Casualty/Disaster Situations

One thumbnail definition of a medical disaster is when the available medical resources are overwhelmed by the demand. By definition then, there are more patients than can be dealt with using traditional care models. Strategies to evaluate large numbers of victims quickly have included the use of prognostic indicators such as elevated heart rate have had limited success (Ritchie *et al.*, 2006). Observation of current level of function and the psychiatric interview remain our most effective tools.

The psychiatrist in the mass casualty situation will quickly become overwhelmed if wedded to a rigid traditional psychiatric interview style. There are simply too many people who have been affected, too few providers, and too little time. Generally, in mass casualty settings, the psychiatrist is asked to do more than assess current symptoms. The clinician is also asked to predict risk for compromised future functioning. A further challenge is that the distress displayed by the patient in the immediate aftermath of the trauma may not correspond well with his or her previous and ultimate level of functioning.

The majority of people experiencing a trauma will exhibit only mild or transitory symptoms. The rate of posttraumatic stress disorder (PTSD) following a traumatic event is highly variable. Rates as low as 10% can be found in the victims of accidents, while 46% of women and 65% of men who have been raped will meet criteria for PTSD (Kessler *et al.*, 1995). Although PTSD is intimately associated with disasters, it is not the only psychiatric disorder seen after a trauma. A significant number of people will develop depressive or anxiety symptoms, but most people will ultimately do well following the trauma (Ursano *et al.*, 1995).

A complicating factor during the posttrauma interview is that it may occur in a variety of nontraditional settings such as homes, shelters, and temporary facilities. One common strategy among military mental health providers is to triage by walking around, the idea being that it is more helpful to interview victims in their own environment than to wait until they venture into the mental health services area. This walking triage may be especially important as at-risk populations include more than just the identified victims of trauma. The psychiatrist in a mass casualty situation should also attend to the distress and functioning of coworkers. They are often the victims of secondary traumatization and provider fatigue. Depending on the size and location of the disaster, the psychiatrist too might have been personally affected. If the clinician has missing friends or relatives or has potentially lost his or her home, his or her ability to evaluate patients might be impacted (Ritchie and Hamilton, 2004).

The interview will be further complicated by the patient's complex and shifting response to the recent trauma. He or she may have intense and mixed emotions regarding the event. There will of course be grief and loss. He or she may also be afraid to remember details of the event. Often there is tremendous anger directed toward people whom he or she holds responsible for the trauma or for a lack of a prompt effective response to the trauma. Guilt about behavior during or after the event is common. He or she may feel that his or her response was inadequate. There also might be guilt about having survived when others did not. All of these make it difficult for casualty survivors to openly discuss the event with the psychiatrist (Connor *et al.*, 2006).

Cultural considerations are always important during the assessment following trauma. Allowing mental health providers of different cultural backgrounds to assist in the aftermath of a trauma may be met with resistance. Since culture may alter how patients express their symptoms, overreliance on DSM phenomenology may be unhelpful. For example, it has been noted following traumas in Japan that the Japanese may be reluctant to acknowledge "depression" even when they meet criteria for it (Connor *et al.*, 2006). In many rural settings, personal identity is bound inextricably to religious identity. Also, a deep attachment to a village may intensify the sense of loss even when personal, household loss has not occurred. All of these cultural factors may impact how the trauma is experienced by the individual (Bryant and Njenga, 2006).

Guidelines for interviewing the victims of mass casualty situations include:

- Look for life-threatening physical conditions. These must be addressed immediately.
- Assess mental status and level of consciousness as these may be indicators of physical injuries or worsening medical conditions.
- Be aware of your appearance and presentation. The psychiatrist will inevitably be seen as an outsider but needs to dress in a fashion that will promote acceptance as a benevolent authority figure by the injured population (Ritchie and Hamilton, 2004).
- Educate survivors regarding normal cognitive, emotional, behavioral, and physical changes following trauma. Highlight that these are common responses to abnormal situations and will likely resolve without specific interventions. Emphasize that these symptoms are not inherently dangerous or an indication of moral or mental weakness.
    - Common impairment includes:
        - *Cognitive* – Memory loss, anomia, impaired decision-making, poor concentration
        - *Emotional* – Anxiety, grief, irritability, feeling overwhelmed, fear of future loss
        - *Behavioral* – Insomnia, hypervigilance, crying, ritualistic behaviors
        - *Physical* – Fatigue, nausea, tremor, motor tics, dizziness, gastrointestinal distress (Flynn and Norwood, 2004; Ritchie *et al.*, 2006; Ursano *et al.*, 2003)
- Watch for symptoms of extreme avoidance, numbing, or dissociations. The presence of dissociations in particular has been associated with an increased risk of PTSD (Ursano *et al.*, 2003).
- *Ask the Victims about the Meaning of the Disaster* – The trauma frequently threatens more than the individual's life, family, or livelihood. Often these events will challenge the victims' understanding of how the world functions. Individuals living with a "just world hypothesis", where good things happen to good people and bad things happen to bad people may find that point of view inadequate to explain what they have just experienced. Others will have their core religious and spiritual beliefs challenged in a way that it had not been challenged before.

- *The Use of Screening Tools* – There is some controversy as to the utility of screening tools, with some authors finding it a useful means to getting information on people quickly and others doubting the reliability of the information obtained (Connor *et al.*, 2006; Ritchie and Hamilton, 2004).
- *Emphasize Strength, Resilience, and Growth* – While the psychiatrist should not minimize the destruction and distress caused by the disaster, it is also important to recognize that these traumatic events are often a time for growth. Individuals will demonstrate strength and coping abilities that they may not have realized that they had. Communities will often pull together and support each other. This growth may not be evident during the initial interview, but the psychiatrist can lay the groundwork for recognizing it by inquiring about it even in the early stages of the post-disaster period.

Summary of Recommendations

- Be prepared to leave the clinic and interview victims where they are.
- Discuss common emotional, physical, and behavioral responses to trauma.
- Watch for cultural differences in responding to trauma.
- Emphasize strength and resilience.

Psychiatric Interview in Special Patient Populations

Even when the psychiatric interview takes place in the comfort of the psychiatrist's office, there can be groups of people who raise special challenges. In general, these are patients whose baseline functioning or illness inherently complicate the interview process. Often adopting a different style or using different questions to elicit data is vital.

Special Populations – Patients with Psychosis

Psychotic symptoms can be divided into those which affect the content of thought and those which alter the flow or form of thought processes. Although routine for psychiatrists, each of these categories presents separate problems for the interviewer. Problems with thought content include delusions, thought blocking, thought insertion, and perceptual abnormalities such as hallucinations. These experiences, which diverge greatly from common experience, make it difficult for these patients to express what is going on in their lives. They may have difficulty putting their fears or belief systems into words. They may have difficulty differentiating events in their lives from internal experiences, which appear to be just as real. Formal thought disorders result in communication that is difficult to follow. Because of loosened associations or incomplete ideas, the interviewer may have trouble getting a coherent story. The interviewer's challenge is to overcome these obstacles and get as much useful information as can be obtained within a reasonable period of time.

Often seriously impaired patients have a long history of psychiatric illness. The psychiatrist during the initial interview should inquire about past interactions with mental health providers. "What should I know about your illness?" "How can I help you?" "What has worked in the past?" "What have other providers tried that did not work?" These past experiences can shape the current interaction (MacKinnon *et al.*, 2006). Positive interactions should be highlighted as evidence of the help that psychiatry can offer. Negative experiences can be acknowledged, followed closely by a description of how this encounter can be different.

There are some strategies that apply to patients with both types of psychotic symptoms. These patients have often been brought for evaluation by someone else and therefore might get frustrated because they are in the hospital. The psychiatrist can sympathize with their resentment during the interview but also note their desire to help the patient. Psychotic symptoms often create a gap between the experience of the patient and of anyone trying to communicate with him or her. This makes it harder to generate empathy for the patient and leaves the provider more likely to do a perfunctory assessment (MacKinnon *et al.*, 2006). To help bridge the gap, the psychiatrist should ask about the symptoms that bother the patient. Perhaps he or she is not bothered by the voices that he or she hears but is upset at feeling constantly tired. Other common complaints might include anxiety, pain, nausea, or problems with sadness. By focusing initially on these symptoms, the provider might be able to bridge some of the gap separating the patient's world from his or her own (Shea, 1988).

- *Example* – A 28-year-old man with a history of schizophrenia is brought into the ED after he was found wandering in a city park by the police. He perseverates on comments such as "I shouldn't be here. I need to go". The psychiatrist perceiving this agitation says: "Some people were pretty concerned that you were getting confused. They have asked me to see if I can help figure out what is going on. You look pretty worried. Is there anything I can help with?"
- *Psychotic Thought Content* – Often the patient is terrified and confused by what he or she is experiencing and might have no reason to believe that the psychiatrist can be of any help. Although the psychiatrist's ability to empathically enter the patient's world can be limited, a therapeutic alliance must be forged (e.g., "Can you help me understand what is upsetting you?"). As is true in any patient encounter, the psychiatrist uses his or her emotional response to what the patient is describing as an important vehicle to enhance communication. Attentiveness to a patient's emotional state can help focus the patient and develop rapport (MacKinnon *et al.*, 2006). There is a need to look for any topic that appears to carry a significant emotional valence since this displays interest in the patient and facilitates clarification of his or her inner experience. With expressions of fear comes the opportunity to offer realistic but consistent hopefulness while emphasizing the current level of safety (Shea, 1988).
    - *Example* – A disheveled 34-year-old woman, Alice, is brought into the ED by the police. She had been arrested running down the street striking cars with a rock. She appears terrified in the ED and is curled into a near fetal position without acknowledging the psychiatrist when he enters. "Alice, you look very upset. Can you tell me what is going on". Alice responds: "I can't take it anymore". She is no longer sure who is harassing her. She figured that by striking the cars she would draw out the assassins who were following her. "Alice, it must be terrible to feel that frightened all of the time. Do you feel safe in here?"

With these few simple sentences, the psychiatrist has made an effort to establish an empathic connection. Demonstrating sympathy for her troubles, the clinician has also addressed her with respect and dignity. These can be the first steps toward developing a meaningful therapeutic rapport.

With a patient who focuses on a single issue, such as a systematic delusion, the psychiatrist will emphasize the need to gain understanding into other aspects of the patient's life. This type of patient will often lose the point of open-ended questions and shift the topic back to the thought that consumes him or her. To get useful information in this case, the psychiatrist will have to shift from open-ended questions to more direct questions. Sometimes these will have to be questions that can be answered by a "yes" or "no".

As in any patient encounter, honesty is vital. Attempts to enhance the therapeutic relationship through misinformation (pretending to see or hear his or her hallucinations or acknowledging conspiracies) are prone to failure. Once the patient realizes that the psychiatrist has not been truthful, the therapeutic alliance is almost certainly damaged, sometimes beyond repair. It is usually possible to accept the patient's response to his or her experiences without agreeing to his or her perception. "I know that you are hearing an evil threatening voice, but I do not hear it and no one else here is hearing it. I think that voice is coming from within your mind".

Other specific advice includes:

- *Delusions* – Realize that you will not be able to convince the patient to abandon his or her delusions, and that he or she will refuse to accept facts that you hold to be incontrovertible. Acknowledge that he or she believes what he or she is telling you and that he or she believes there is abundant evidence supporting him or her. Do not hesitate, however, to wonder with him or her if there might be some other way to explain the facts. The psychiatrist can acknowledge the anxiety and frustration the patient experiences in trying to convince others to believe something that they know to be true (MacKinnon *et al.*, 2006).
- *Paranoia* – Interviewing the paranoid patient is one of the most difficult challenges for the psychiatrist. This patient will mistrust motives from the start. He or she will present himself or herself in a guarded fashion based on his or her fear that what he or she says will be used to hurt him or her. Tactful telling of the truth in these situations may not win the patient over but is still the psychiatrist's best option. Acknowledge that he or she is not free to leave when he or she wants and that your evaluation will play a role in what happens to him or her. "You might disagree, but I think the people who brought you here are truly concerned for your safety. They want me to help determine if you are safe". Avoid humor with these patients. They are unlikely to enjoy it and can easily assume that you are making fun of them, thereby increasing their agitation. The psychiatrist will often agree with the facts that the patient presents without agreeing with his or her interpretation of those facts. "I believe that you saw five black cars pass by your house. I am just not sure that means that the CIA has you under surveillance". Resist the patient's attempt to pull you into a power struggle. The goal is to assess his or her functioning and safety, not to debate with him or her. Regardless of good intentions and efforts, the patient may be suspicious of the psychiatrist or even contemptuous. Accept his or her need for emotional distance and psychological defenses while proceeding with the interview (MacKinnon *et al.*, 2006).

- *Hallucinations* – The voices that the patient hears and the things that he or she sees are just as real to him or her as you are. Therefore, attempts to dismiss them or minimize their importance will rarely succeed. Instead, ask about them as you would about any other experience (Shea, 1988). You can ask for details such as:
  - How many voices are you hearing?
  - What are they saying?
  - What can you tell me about them?
  - Do they remind you of anyone you know?
  - Are they talking with you now?
  - How difficult is it for you to pay attention to me with them talking?
- *Formal Thought Disorder* – These patients are attempting to express themselves but are unable to do so in a fashion that can be followed by the psychiatrist. The psychiatrist will usually pick up on this within the first few minutes of conversation. Readily, but tactfully, admit to difficulty understanding what the patient is trying to say. This can usually be done without humiliating or blaming the patient. The psychiatrist might find open-ended questioning as being unproductive. Attempts to gain information through direct questioning should nevertheless include reflections on the patient's spontaneous speech and topics of conversation. This presents the best opportunity for making an empathic connection with the patient.
- *Example* – A 45-year-old man with psychotic mania has extremely loosened associations. His rambling digressions include his involvement with both the president and the governor and their plans for him to assist them personally on special projects. As he is completing the interview, the psychiatrist comments: "I know I have not heard about everything that is going on in your life, but listening to you for these few minutes I am struck by the sense that you have a lot of potential and opportunities, but are not quite sure what you want from your life".

Summary of Recommendations

- Ask about past interactions with mental health.
- Show empathy for their distress.
- Acknowledge their perceptions without necessarily agreeing with their conclusions.
- Do not debate with them.

Special Populations – Suicidal Patients

Patients with a significant risk of suicide are an extremely common cause of emergent psychiatric consultations. The psychiatrist often enters the situation with little to no previous alliance with the patient. In order to obtain useful and truthful information, the psychiatrist must quickly establish a working rapport. Since suicidality is the reason for the consult, there is a temptation to jump immediately into a discussion of that issue. The patient, however, has little motivation to be honest with a provider he or she is just meeting. If he or she is truly suicidal, he or she will see it in his or her best interest to be deceptive. If he or she is not suicidal, he or she will either tell the truth, which might make it difficult to distinguish him or her from the deceitful suicidal patient, or he or she might try to deceive the provider for other reasons such as an attempt to gain admission to the hospital.

The best strategy for the psychiatrist is to spend some time getting to know the patient broadly before broaching the topic of suicidality. This discussion will help build rapport but will also start filling in the suicide risk factors that are central to the assessment.

- What has brought them into the hospital?
- What do they think can be done to help them?
- Ask about their recent stresses: What has changed in your life recently?
- Ask about recent neurovegetative symptoms.
- Ask about their past psychiatric history: Have they ever been admitted for psychiatric reasons? Have they ever been treated as an outpatient?
- Are they currently under the care of a mental health professional?
- Ask about their social support.

After gathering this background information, the psychiatrist can move onto more direct questions. Normalizing thoughts of death and suicide is often an effective means of starting the exploration of those issues, e.g., "Many people in your situation would have thoughts of death. They might wish they were dead or have thoughts about killing themselves. Have you had thoughts like those?"

The psychiatrist will need to ask about suicidality directly.

- *Suicidal Ideation* – How frequent are the thoughts of killing themselves? How long have they been present? Are they changing in intensity or frequency?
- *Suicidal Plan* – Do they have a specific plan to end their life? Is it realistic? Is it lethal? Are they likely to be rescued in the attempt?
- *Suicidal Intent* – Do they want to die? Do they feel it is inevitable that they will die?
- *Preparation and Rehearsal for Suicide* – Have they obtained lethal means? Have they practiced the suicide attempt?
- *Suicide Attempts* – Have they ever tried to kill themselves in the past? Do they have family or friends who have committed suicide?
- *Protective Factors* – We should also ask about what has kept them alive to this point.

The risk assessment, however, includes more than just questions asked to the patient. The interviewer's observational skills are also necessary. What is the patient's affect? Does he or she maintain good eye contact? Does he or she display psychomotor retardation? Is there significant anxiety or agitation?

Gathering this information is only the first part of the suicide risk assessment. Once the information has been gathered, the clinician should consider the patient's acute and chronic risk of suicide. It might be helpful to divide these risk factors into several categories: static risk factors, dynamic risk factors, and warning signs.

- Static risk factors for suicide are often demographic information that cannot be quickly altered.
  - *Male Sex* – Men are three to four times more likely to commit suicide.
  - *Age* – Although there are legitimate concerns about suicide in young adults, in general the rate of population is highest among the oldest individuals.

  - *Race* – Elevated rates of suicide are found in White and Native Americans than in Black and Hispanic Americans.
  - Family history of suicide.
  - *Prior Suicide Attempts* – This is perhaps the most robust risk factor. Approximately 10–15% of those who have attempted suicide will ultimately kill themselves.
  - *Being Single* – Although it is not found in every study, being divorced, widowed, or never married seems to increase the risk of suicide.
- Dynamic risk factors for suicide are ones that can be changed through intervention.
  - Untreated mental illness.
  - *Emotional Turmoil* – This can be brought on by recent financial or legal problems, acute and chronic medical conditions, or relationship issues.
  - Expressed suicidality.
  - Access to weapons and other lethal means.
- Warning signs are indicators that suicide may be imminent and are further divided into two tiers. Both of these groups still indicate marked elevation of risk but the second is more concerning.
  - Warning signs include hopelessness, rage, anger, acting recklessly, feeling trapped, increasing alcohol or drug use, withdrawal from friends, anxiety, agitation, altered sleep, dramatic changes in mood, and seeing no reason for living.
  - Imminent warning signs include direct threats to harm themselves, searching for means to kill themselves, and writing or talking about death and dying.

The key for thorough suicide risk assessment and management is to incorporate all of the elicited information and then generate a comprehensive plan based on it. The plan should minimize as many dynamic factors and warning signs as possible while enhancing the protective factors. This should be done in a biopsychosocial manner. Biologic interventions can include starting antidepressants, realizing that these may take several weeks to take effect and might even increase agitation in the short term. If insomnia has been a significant factor, then the psychiatrist can consider safe methods for assisting sleep. Psychological interventions should include the initiation of psychotherapy, which can be facilitated during the initial interview by delineating some of the major conflicts that are upsetting the patient. Social interactions can include increasing support as well as helping to create a safer environment for the patient. Environmental manipulation can include reducing access to lethal means of self-harm. Often with the patient's permission, family and friends can be involved in controlling access to potentially dangerous weapons and medications. Social manipulation might also involve hospitalization as a means of protecting the patient while waiting for the other interventions to have an opportunity to work (Welton, 2007). Providers can never completely prevent suicide in patients who have committed themselves to dying, but a thorough evaluation and appropriate intervention is the best method for helping these patients.

Summary of Recommendations

- Work to establish rapport.
- Be aware of and inquire about suicide risk factors.
- Ask about protective factors.
- Biopsychosocial interventions should target dynamic risk factors and warning signs.

Special Populations – Children/Adolescents

Alterations in interview style and content must be expected when working with children and adolescents. Even within this group, there is great variation depending on the age and maturational level of the child and the circumstances leading to the interview. The interview of a depressed or traumatized 5-year-old will be very different than the interview of a depressed or traumatized 9-year-old.

Adults will usually enter a psychiatrist's office with some idea of the role and capabilities of a psychiatrist. The child may not have this understanding and may find the experience extremely foreign and threatening. Helping to clarify children's expectation about the interview and their perspective on the issues that brought them in to be assessed is a good starting point. Especially with younger children, it is helpful to clarify that they are not in trouble and have not been brought in because they are bad (Sadock and Sadock, 2003).

The psychiatrist might want to start the interview with a review of the less charged aspects of the child's life such as involvement in hobbies, sports, and favorite leisure time activities. These topics also provide useful information about the number and quality of his or her interactions and social, academic, and physical development (Sadock and Sadock, 2003). Younger, school-age children can be brought into a room with a variety of toys and observed in unstructured play. As the child plays, the interviewer can ask questions about the child's inner life. Having toys that are reminiscent of home situations (e.g., adult and child dolls) can also lead to fruitful discussions about relationships with the child, inevitably conveying information about his or her home life. Another useful technique is to ask the child to draw. Asking children to draw family members and having them talk about their families can also establish their views on family dynamics. The interviewer looks for themes or patterns in the child's play and drawings. There are still questions that need to be asked, but the psychiatrist will likely need to modify the questions. Open-ended questions may be less successful than giving the child several possible answers. The interviewer can still try an open-ended question but have a list of possible answers if the child cannot answer (Sadock and Sadock, 2003).

- *Example* – During an interview the child is asked, "How have you been feeling?" She answers, "Good I guess". The interviewer goes on, "Have you been feeling sad or angry or scared?"

Some of the differences in interview technique are straightforward and require sensitivity to developmentally appropriate language. The simple question "Are you depressed" may have no meaning to a bright 8-year-old, or even worse, may mean something completely different than what the clinician intended. Often simple behavioral or functional questions can be substituted for more complex or abstract ones. Rather than asking about lethargy, anhedonia, appetite, and anxiety, the interviewer can ask questions such as: "Do you get tired easier than your friends?", "What do you do with your friends that is really fun?", "Do you eat everything on your plate at meals?", or "Is there anything that is scaring you?" In addition to ascertaining the DSMIV-TR criteria for mental illness, the interviewer working with small children should also attempt to obtain an understanding of their level of development. This will help guide future interventions if deficits are found.

One model used to understand the development of younger children is the Developmental, Individual difference, Relationship (DIR) model. This model seeks to facilitate a comprehensive understanding of the child through a systematic evaluation of three major components of his or her mental life. The interviewer examines the functional emotional development of the child, the sensory reactivity/cognitive processing/executive functioning of the child, and finally the relationships the child has with significant caregivers in his or her life.

- *Functional Emotional Development* – The first category involves the child's ability to work toward emotionally meaningful goals. This will be evaluated by looking at a variety of responses and behaviors:
    - Is the child able to retain a sense of calm while watching and listening to his or her caregivers?
    - Does the child display apparent pleasure from his or her interactions with his or her caregiver?
    - Does the child engage in reciprocal communication with the others?
    - Can the child engage in problem-solving communication?
    - Can the child engage in creative and imaginative play?
    - Can the child give meaning to symbols?
    - Can the child display the ability to use logic, reality testing, and judgment in interactions with others?
- Sensory reactivity, cognitive processing, and executive functioning are also assessed. This category recognizes the fact that even children who have significant similarities in their emotional development may have significant differences in their cognitive function. These variations can be the result of genetic, prenatal, or maturational factors. The areas to be evaluated include:
    - Reactivity to sensory perception
        - Does the child underreact or overreact to sensory stimuli?
    - Sensory processing
        - Is the child able to register, decode, and comprehend what he or she is hearing and seeing?
    - Ability to process and react to affect with action or communication
        - Does the child understand emotional responses and act accordingly?
    - Ability to plan behavior and predict consequences of behavior
- Assessing the style and quality of relationships
    - Does the child have appropriate interactions with primary caregivers and family members?
    - How does the child choose to engage with his or her environment? Does he or she seek out interactions with those around him or her? Does he or she explore his or her surroundings appropriately?

The DIR model leads to an individualized profile of the child that can serve as a basis for developing targeted interventions. It considers biological and psychological development as well as valuing the social interactions as a significant factor in child growth (Greenspan and Wieder, 2003).

A one-on-one interview of the child is rarely sufficient to develop a complete understanding of his or her world and mental state. Children often lack the self-observing functions necessary to describe themselves in an objective fashion. The younger the child, the fewer his or her reference points for normal behavior. Because of these factors, collateral information is vital. Parents or other primary caretakers can provide the best overview of the child and can provide key insights into the developmental history. In addition to augmenting the child's perspective, these caregivers can discuss neurovegetative symptoms such as eating and sleeping habits as well as describe interactions with others (family and friends). If possible, both parents should be interviewed. This will sometimes help provide a more balanced perspective as well as clarifying the differing expectations, perceptions, and roles that exist within the family.

In addition to family information, with school-age children, information from teachers and counselors can be extremely important. The classroom represents a ready-made control group where the child's performance and behavior can be directly compared to those of peers. Parents may at times have a very skewed view of their child based on their personal expectations and what they see at home. Experienced teachers and school counselors often have a more accurate view of the child's functioning in structured and controlled settings.

As the interview proceeds, the issue of confidentiality can be introduced. Confidentiality will depend largely on the age and developmental stage of the child. With very young children, there will be very little that will be held back from the parents. As the child ages, he or she will have more right to maintain some information from his or her parents (Sadock and Sadock, 2003).

Often parents wish to be present when the psychiatrist talks with their child. Children may also find the doctor's office an intimidating place and wish strongly that their parents stay with them. In both of these instances, the interviewer should politely push to be alone with the child for at least part of the interview. One common strategy is to speak with the child and parents at first. This gives the parents and child an opportunity to help define the problem. It is also a helpful time to ask about past treatment, past similar experiences, and trends in symptoms. Hopefully, by this time, both the child and parents are feeling more comfortable with the psychiatrist, who can then outline the rest of the interview process. After speaking to the parents and child, most psychiatrists will prefer to speak privately with the child. This will be followed by interviewing the parents and then bringing everyone back into the room.

Interviewing the child without his or her parents provides several advantages. In addition to increasing disclosure from the child, it allows the interviewer greater freedom to conduct the interview without having to explain interview techniques or involve the parents in the conversation. It also keeps the parents from answering for their child and solidifies the relationship with the child. Speaking to the parents alone similarly helps them to reveal information about the child and their home life that they may not feel comfortable expressing in front of the child. Finally, bringing everyone back into the room for a few minutes will allow the psychiatrist some additional insight into the family's functioning. How does the child interact with his or her parents? Does he or she turn to the parents as a source of support? Is he or she dependent on the parents to speak for him or her? How does the child's interaction with the psychiatrist change when his or her parents come back into the room? Bringing the family back together also allows the psychiatrist to ensure that all know what the treatment plan includes and what the next step will be.

Adolescent Issues – During the interview of adolescents, the psychiatrist must remember that their inner world and experiences might be much broader than their parents realize, and, therefore, nothing can be assumed. The interviewer must ask teenagers about their sexual experiences, alcohol consumption, and recreational drug use. If these experiences are normalized, there is a greater chance of getting truthful information from the adolescent, e.g., "Many teens your age have already had sexual experiences. What experiences have you had?" As teens may feel uncomfortable answering these issues in front of their parents, interviewing them separately is crucial. They may still be hesitant to answer questions if confidentiality has not already been discussed.

The interview of a minor carries with it legal as well as ethical obligations to ensure the safety of the child. This can include inquiring about abuse or neglect as well as asking questions about violence at school, in the neighborhood, and at home. Particular interest should be paid to the issue of punishment for misbehavior. Most states will have a requirement that a reasonable suspicion of abuse must be reported to state agencies for further evaluation.

Summary of Recommendations

- Clarify interview process with child and parents.
- Inquire about all aspects of child's life.
- Interview child and parents alone and together.
- Consider developmental issues.
- Discuss confidentiality.

Special Populations – Using Interpreters

An increasingly common situation is when the patient and psychiatrist are separated by language. Subtleties of speech and nonverbal communication are central in understanding patients. Differences in language between the patient and interviewer can obfuscate those vital clues. Even slight problems with fluency can have a significant impact. Studies have found that psychoanalysis conducted with bilingual people is more successful in their first language than in their second (Farooq and Fear, 2003). Most facilities have made some accommodations for dealing with patients who do not speak English, but working with these interpreters does not eliminate all of the challenges. There are several categories of interpreters that might be used. These include family members or friends, bilingual hospital personnel, or outside volunteers/contractors. Each category has potential risks and benefits.

Family/Friends

One of the primary advantages to using family is availability. Often they will already be nearby when the psychiatrist arrives. Becoming interpreters provides them an opportunity to directly help the patient. Their involvement also contributes to the patient's support of the treatment plan since very meaningful people have been involved in the discussion. Another advantage is that family and friends may have a wealth of knowledge about the patient's biopsychosocial history. Often they are familiar with the patient's medical history and current medications. They can provide instant collateral information. If the patient is being unclear, evasive, or deceitful, they may share this observation with the clinician. They can also comment on changes that they have seen in the patient over time. The psychiatrist can ask if the patient is expressing himself or herself as he or she normally does. "Does he or she sound confused or appear nervous or sad?" Despite the advantages of using family and friends, however, the disadvantages may be even greater.

If the psychiatrist does not know the patient, then he or she probably does not know the family either. The interviewer will be unaware of who in the family knows the patient well and who will be the most truthful. There is a temptation for the family member to change the story to protect the good name of the family through excluding or minimizing embarrassing information as he or she translates (Phelan and Parkman, 1995). Family members may have preconceived ideas about the patient's condition. They can steer the psychiatrist in a way to cast blame on who or what they think is responsible for the patient's distress. Family members without medical training or background may not understand the questions that the interviewer is asking, but may be hesitant to ask for clarification. On the other hand, they may not understand the patient's response and rather than report the patient's distorted information, they may insert their own answer to the question. They, of course, might be providing accurate information, but at this stage in the assessment, the interviewer needs to hear the patient's responses in an unadulterated form. There is also no control over the quality and nature of the relationship that the patient has with the family members. Perhaps the family member who is volunteering to translate is being abusive or neglectful toward the patient, and this may not be clear during the interview. Ideally, family members should provide a calming experience for the patient, yet often the closest relationships can be the most provocative. This can lead to increased agitation during the interview. Family members may be more likely than other interpreters to insert their own questions and openly disagree with the patient's answers to questions (Phelan and Parkman, 1995). Privacy is also a significant concern since the patient is asked to disclose highly personal information in front of individuals with whom he or she is likely to interact throughout his or her lifetime.

Bilingual Staff

Many psychiatrists prefer to rely on their bilingual staff members, especially if these are mental health workers. These individuals will be knowledgeable about their role as interpreters. Appreciating colloquialisms and common expressions facilitates the interviewer's intentions and meanings in ways that are preferable to a literal word-for-word translation. The patient may be relieved to have a staff member with whom he or she can talk freely and will often turn to them for support. This supportive presence may encourage the patient to be more honest and disclosing. Because these interpreters are trained medical personnel, the interviewer is often more comfortable in inquiring into sensitive issues. Questions about drug and alcohol use, sexual tendencies, and infidelities may be difficult to ask when using a family interpreter, but will be significantly easier when the interpreter is a medical professional.

These trained staff members can describe basic mental functions such as thought processes and thought content. "Does the patient ramble?", "Is the patient answering questions logically?", and "Is he or she paying attention to the conversation?" are questions that can be answered with reasonable certainty by these medically knowledgeable interpreters.

Despite these advantages, there are some drawbacks in using bilingual staff members. Since they might be trained in mental health interviewing, they may change the question from the one asked to one they think should have been asked. Their judgment may be accurate, but it adds a complicating factor to the interview as the interviewer will not know if the patient is being evasive, is uncertain of the answer, or was simply not asked the intended question. Since these translators are more familiar with mental health language, they may tend to paraphrase a patient's answers, thereby complicating the assessment of the patient's use of language.

- *Example* – A psychiatrist is interviewing a patient using a mental health technician as an interpreter. The psychiatrist asks if the patient is having any trouble sleeping. The technician speaks for quite a while. The patient gives a brief response and the technician replies: "She does not have any neurovegetative symptoms". Unless this psychiatrist goes back to clarify the exact symptoms, it will be unclear which symptoms were asked about and which were not.

Another issue with hospital personnel is the assumption that all speakers of a language can understand each other equally well. The reality is far different. Spanish speakers taught continental Spanish may have some difficulty understanding a Spanish speaker from rural Columbia. An American may have a similar problems understanding a Scot from Glasgow. Not only are the accents sometimes difficult to understand, but local idioms may be hard to follow.

Remote Interpreters

Many hospitals have turned to the services of paid interpreters who are accessed by phone. The interviewer is in the room with the patient while both are speaking through an interpreter in some distant location. Many of these interpreters are extremely fluent in multiple languages and proficient at their jobs. They have been instructed to ask questions in as close to a word-to-word translation as possible and to convey the answers in a similar fashion. Because they are used to consulting to medical facilities, they are adept at employing medical terms as well as making normal conversation. Since they do not know the patient, they have little bias and can relate responses in a straightforward fashion. When asked, these interpreters can give comments about the patient's use of language and ability to express themselves. They can be asked simple questions about the patient's speech such as "Were they easy to understand?" and "Did they answer the questions appropriately?"

The fact that the interpreter is not in the room, however, adds uncertainty to the translation. Assessing nonverbal cues may be problematic. The interpreter may have difficulty understanding tone and inflection over the phone lines. Although the interviewer has every reason to trust the interpreter, the patient may not choose to do so. If the patient is suspicious of the interpreter, he or she tends to be less disclosing and more evasive. When it comes to asking potentially uncomfortable personal questions, the remote trained professional is generally more comfortable than a family member but less comfortable than the bilingual coworker.

The push toward brevity is a common problem when utilizing an interpreter. The use of a translator often places the interviewer and the patient in an unfamiliar and uncomfortable circumstance. In addition, the interview often takes much longer than usual. Both the patient and psychiatrist may grow weary of the long pauses and delays in communication. The interviewer may get frustrated with the struggle to get answers for his or her questions. All of these factors may lead the psychiatrist to prematurely terminate the assessment, thereby relying on a minimum of information and/or making unwarranted assumptions. An interpreter may also have a tendency to condense information in an attempt to be more efficient. The interpreter may take the interview's open-ended questions and change them to quicker, close-ended questions, falsely giving the interviewer the idea of limited spontaneous speech by the patient (Farooq and Fear, 2003). The patient may also try to speed up the process by deliberately shortening his or her answers so that he or she will be understood more quickly. This deprives the psychiatrist of an accurate view of the patient's inner world and experiences. All of these can lead to subpar interviews and patient care. The psychiatrist can guard against this by allotting more time than usual for the interview and acknowledging the patient's frustration with the process.

The clinician should meet with the interpreter before the interview to explain the purpose of the interview and to clarify the anticipated questions. If the interpreter has questions about the medical terms being used, these can be addressed prior to meeting with the patient. Further, the importance of word-by-word interpretation and the importance of discerning evidence of a formal thought disorder, neologisms, or hallucinations can be emphasized. If possible, using the same interpreter on subsequent interviews promotes continuity and rapport (Phelan and Parkman, 1995).

After introductions, the psychiatrist will review the role of the interpreter and the mandate of confidentiality. With marginally fluent, English-speaking patients, the interviewer should suggest that an interpreter be brought in. Patients who have good conversational English may find themselves stymied by the demands of a psychiatric interview. Patients may be embarrassed by their limited grasp of the language and might provide answers to what they think was asked rather than request clarification. The interpreter standing nearby gives them another alternative for handling this situation (Phelan and Parkman, 1995).

During the interview, it is important for the interviewer to look at the patient even while the patient responds directly to the interpreter. In employing a remote interpreter, there can be a tendency to look at either the loudspeaker or phone while waiting for answers. This emphasizes the separation between the patient and the interviewer, however, and should be avoided. Observing the patient while he or she speaks also permits the psychiatrist to view nonverbal communications such as affect and mannerisms.

The interviewer should speak at a slightly slower than normal rate but still try to maintain a natural pace and rhythm. The interpreter will sometimes rely on inflection and rhythm of the interviewer to help set the inflection and rhythm of his or her questions. The interviewer should not ask multipart, ambiguous, or complex questions as they often confuse the interpreter and/or the patient.

- *Example* – "Do you have problems with sleep, and if you do, is that a problem getting to sleep, staying asleep, or with waking the next morning?" This inquiry should be broken down into a series of simple, direct questions starting with the open-ended question "Tell me about your sleeping".

One other specific issue involves the use of sign language. In those cases, the interpreter should be situated beside or slightly behind the interviewer so the patient can watch the interviewer's lips but then move quickly to the signer's hands (Phelan and Parkman, 1995).

Summary of Recommendations

- Use trained medical interpreters whenever possible.
- Ask for word-by-word translation.
- Ask the interpreter about the patient's thought processes.
- Allow for more time than usual.
- Focus on the patient during the interview.

Special Populations – Cross-cultural Issues

Working in a multicultural arena presents a constant challenge for the psychiatrist. Often the same words may have remarkably different meanings for each of the parties requiring additional time to explore issues thoughtfully. Stereotyping and personal biases dramatically alter any clinical relationship. Assumptions about shared experiences are to be avoided.

- *Example* – Both the therapist and the patient grew up as Latinas in a southwestern region of the country. As had been the case for the interviewer, there was an assumption that the church was a central and comforting part of the patient's life. Later, it becomes apparent that the church is united in the patient's mind with her autocratic demanding and abusive father.

Special Population – Telepsychiatry

In an effort to enhance psychiatric coverage to rural and isolated locations, many health systems are turning to telepsychiatry, which allows psychiatric evaluation from a distant location. This is part of an overall increase in the use of information technology to enhance medical care. According to the American Telemedicine Association, 20 million Americans get some part of their health care remotely (Ravn, 2012). Patients who would not be able to see specialists in person can still receive their care through video links to their Primary Care Provider's office.

In addition to reaching isolated populations, another potential advantage of telepsychiatry is cost savings. While purchasing and maintaining the computer and camera equipment at the base location and distant sites can be a significant upfront cost, this will likely be offset by the savings that comes from not having to pay the psychiatrist's travel expenses. A 6-month study compared in-person treatment of depression with telepsychiatry and found that the per session cost of telepsychiatry was more than that of in-person sessions ($86.16 vs. $63.25). When travel costs were included, however, the cost became equal with a drive of 22 miles. If the psychiatrist had to drive more than 22 miles to the distant site, then telepsychiatry was less expensive (Ruskin *et al.*, 2004). An additional financial benefit comes from an expected increase in the number of patient contacts. As the provider does not lose time driving to the distant site, he or she has more time to see patients.

There is mounting evidence that in addition to being fiscally beneficial, telepsychiatry provides good quality care. When adequate equipment is used, telepsychiatry can accurately assess cognitive functioning, depressive, anxiety, and psychotic symptoms (O'Reilly *et al.*, 2007). A 2005 meta-analysis of 14 studies with 500 patients found no difference in accuracy or patient satisfaction using telepsychiatry versus in-person evaluations (Hyler *et al.*, 2005).

There have been a number of positive trials examining patient outcomes after receiving telepsychiatry services. One hundred and nineteen veterans with depression were followed for 6 months by in-person psychiatry or telepsychiatry. This study found that depressive symptoms, adherence to treatment, drop-out rates, and satisfaction levels were equivalent. When travel expenses were included, the two treatments were equal in costs (Ruskin *et al.*, 2004). A Canadian study tracked 495 patients who were followed in person or by telepsychiatry. After 4 months of treatment, the patients were reassessed, and both groups had similar improvements in symptoms (O'Reilly *et al.*, 2007).

The United States' Veterans Administration (VA) has promoted the use of telemedicine for mental health services since the early 2000s as a means of reaching out to veterans in rural settings. Between 2003 and early 2012, there had been almost 500,000 tele-mental health encounters with 98,609 veterans. The tele-mental health technology used during 2006–2010 allowed for greater access to evaluations, psychotherapy, and psychoeducational programs. The study also examined the use of mental health resources before and after enrollment and found that the number of admissions and hospital days decreased by nearly 25% after patients enrolled in a telepsychiatry program (Godleski *et al.*, 2012). While telepsychiatry undoubtedly presents exciting opportunities to bring psychiatric services to areas that had been neglected, using telepsychiatry to interview patients creates new challenges.

There are legal and privileging issues that are pertinent to telepsychiatry. Can interviews cross state lines? What are the privileging and licensure requirements if they do? What if patients become agitated during the interview? What if they threaten themselves or someone else? How can the interviewing psychiatrist respond when hundreds of miles away? These questions will need to be answered on a case-by-case basis (Monnier *et al.*, 2003).

Some challenges are strictly technical ones. Compatibility of equipment and software and the adequacy of the available bandwidth need to be addressed. As would be expected, the broader the bandwidth and the better the quality of the picture, the more accurate the assessment. Forty-two patients were assessed in person and via telepsychiatry using a standardized rating scale. The telepsychiatry evaluations were conducted using either narrowband or broadband technology. The quality of assessments utilizing broadband technology was similar to face-to-face interviews. Narrowband technology, however, led to inferior assessments. This decrease in accuracy was likely due to poor image quality and the inability to assess nonverbal cues (Yoshino *et al.*, 2001).

With less than optimal technology, the provider may have difficulty conducting numerous parts of the interview. The psychiatrist may have more difficulty assessing tone of voice. Depending on the camera angle, some important nonverbal cues may go unnoticed. If the patient is not speaking into a high-quality microphone, the clinician may have difficulty hearing or understanding the patient. Eye contact is also difficult to establish. Should the psychiatrist and patient look at the picture on the monitor or into the camera? With adequate preparation, however, many of these problems can be solved.

Before beginning an interview, the psychiatrist should become thoroughly acquainted with the functioning and capability of the equipment. He or she can optimize the experience by having an assistant at the distant site play the role of the patient sitting where he or she would sit and speaking in a normal, soft, and then loud tone. This advance work can also include adjusting the camera and the lighting so that the patient's features and upper body are plainly visible. The psychiatrist can also be positioned to look into the camera while still having a good view of the patient on the monitor.

To minimize the risk of agitation or threatened violence, some locations may choose to have a mental health technician or other medical personnel sitting in the room with the patient. Having this third-party in the session may raise issues of confidentiality and may adversely impact the therapeutic alliance. Another solution to these safety concerns is to have a second line that the provider can use to instantly notify the distant site if the patient demonstrates a deteriorating mental state or expresses concerns about harming himself or herself or others.

The provider should speak in a slightly slow but precise fashion. Early in the interview, significant procedures should be reviewed with the patient. What should be done when the connection is lost? What should occur if the image freezes? What would lead the psychiatrist to contact the distant site for assistance? This is in essence a modified informed consent. Repeatedly checking in with patients during the interview regarding their mood and emotional state is critical since appreciation of nonverbal cues is lessened. Feedback from patients about their ability to see, hear, and understand the psychiatrist is essential as the psychiatrist's ability to see, hear, and understand the patient. Since both the patient and interviewer quickly become aware of the limitations of this modality, asking them to lean forward or speak more slowly is a reasonable request to make.

The US Army began a telepsychiatry program linking Walter Reed Army Medical Center in Washington, DC and Carlisle Barracks in Carlisle, Pennsylvania. They assessed patients' initial concerns about using telepsychiatry services and then followed up about the experience. Nearly a third had concerns about privacy issues before starting telepsychiatry, but, after using the service, that number had been cut in half. Those expressing concerns about confidentiality decreased from 76% before using the program to only 4% with some experience. None of the patients thought that the telepsychiatry experience interfered with their relationship with their psychiatrists. Ninety-six percent eventually agreed that they were comfortable using telepsychiatry services and 84% thought that the care they received was as good if not better than if it had been face-to-face (Schneider, 2006). Although telepsychiatry is still relatively young and the data are limited, with proper safeguards, telepsychiatry appears to be an appropriate venue for psychiatric evaluations.

It is as of yet unclear how telepsychiatry impacts the therapeutic alliance. While patients receiving telepsychiatry often report satisfaction with their interactions with their tele-provider, this may be due to increased convenience and their getting to see a specialist than the creation of a positive relationship with the tele-provider (Monnier *et al.*, 2003). Large-scale studies looking specifically at the therapeutic alliance have yet to be done. It has been suggested that the issue of therapeutic alliance using telepsychiatry may be rapidly shifting as younger generations are increasingly comfortable with carrying out intimate relationships via digital connections (Zur, 2012).

Summary of Recommendations

- Use high-quality, broadband equipment.
- Establish procedures for the handling of emergencies and loss of connection.
- Check in with patient frequently about his or her mood and the interview experience.
- Deliberately attempt to enhance the alliance with the patient.

Conclusions

The psychiatric interview is the psychiatrist's chief means of obtaining information about the patient. Every interview is unique. The life history of each patient is always different from every other patient encountered. When the patient and psychiatrist meet, they are at the juxtaposition of a particular time in the life of the patient and the professional and personal life of the psychiatrist. If they had met 3 months earlier or later, the interview might be considerably different. This chapter has looked at some special circumstances, patient populations, and interactions that frequently create additional challenges for the psychiatrist. By attending to the characteristics of the interview setting and the patient's circumstances, the psychiatrist can adapt strategies and techniques to overcome these difficulties and provide excellent patient care.

References

Bryant RA and Njenga FG (2006) Cultural sensitivity: Making trauma assessment and treatment plans culturally relevant. *Journal of Clinical Psychiatry* 67(Suppl. 2), 74–79.

Connor KM, Foa EB and Davidson JRT (2006) Practical assessment and evaluation of mental health problems following a mass disaster. *Journal of Clinical Psychiatry* 67(Suppl. 2), 26–33.

Farooq S and Fear C (2003) Working through interpreters. *Advances in Psychiatric Treatment* 9, 104–109.

Feinstein R and Plutchik R (1990) Violence and suicide risk assessment in the psychiatric emergency room. *Comprehensive Psychiatry* 31, 337–343.

Flynn BW and Norwood A (2004) Defining normal psychological reactions to disaster. *Psychiatric Annals* 34, 597–603.

Godleski L, Darkins A and Peters J (2012) Outcomes of 98,609 U.S. Department of Veterans affairs patients enrolled in Telemental Health Services, 2006–2010. *Psychiatric Services* 63, 383–385.

Greenspan SI and Wieder S (2003) Diagnostic classification in infancy and early childhood, in *Psychiatry*, 2nd edn (eds Tasman A, Kay J and Lieberman JA). John Wiley & Sons, Ltd, Chichester.

Hyler SE, Gangure DP and Batchelder ST (2005) Can telepsychiatry replace in-person psychiatric assessments? A review and meta-analysis of comparison studies. *CNS Spectrum* 10, 403–413.

Kessler RC, Sonnega A, Bromet E *et al.* (1995) Posttraumatic stress disorder in the national comorbidity survey. *Archives of General Psychiatry* 52, 1048–1060.

MacKinnon RA, Michels R and Buckley PJ (2006) *The Psychiatric Interview in Clinical Practice*, 2nd edn. American Psychiatric Publishing Inc., Washington, DC.

Meyers J and Stein S (2000) The psychiatric interview in the emergency department. *Emergency Medicine Clinics of North America* 18, 175–183.

Miller PR (2001) Inpatient diagnostic assessments: 2. Interrater reliability and outcomes of structured vs. unstructured interviews. *Psychiatric Research* 105, 265–271.

Miller PR (2002) Inpatient diagnostic assessments: 3. Causes and effects of diagnostic imprecision. *Psychiatry Research* 111, 191–197.

Miller PR, Dasher R, Collins R *et al.* (2001) Inpatient diagnostic assessments: 1. Accuracy of structured vs. unstructured interviews. *Psychiatry Research* 105, 255–264.

Monnier J, Knapp RG and Frueh BC (2003) Recent advances in telepsychiatry: An updated review. *Psychiatric Services* 54, 1604–1609.

Nichita EC and Buckley PF (2007) Informed consent and competency: Doctor's dilemma on the consultation liaison service. *Psychiatry* 4, 53–55.

O'Reilly R, Bishop J, Maddox K *et al.* (2007) Is telepsychiatry equivalent to face-to-face psychiatry? Results from a randomized controlled equivalence trial. *Psychiatric Service* 58, 836–843.

Perry S and Viederman M (1981a) Adaptation of residents to consultation-liaison psychiatry; II. Working with the nonpsychiatric staff. *General Hospital Psychiatry* 3, 149–156.

Perry S and Viederman M (1981b) Adaptation of residents to consultation-liaison psychiatry; I. Working with the physically ill. *General Hospital Psychiatry* 3, 141–147.

Phelan M and Parkman S (1995) How to do it: Work with an interpreter. *BMJ* 311, 555.

Philbrick KL, Rundell JR, Netzel PJ *et al.* (2012) *Clinical Manual of Psychosomatic Medicine: A Guide to Consultation-Liaison Psychiatry*, 2nd edn. American Psychiatric Publishing Inc., Washington, DC.

Ravn K (2012) Telemedicine means caregivers are remote, but their care isn't. *LA Times*, September 13. http://articles.latimes.com/2012/sep/13/health/la-he-future-of-telemedicine-20120913. Accessed on February 1, 2013.

Ritchie EC and Hamilton SE (2004) Assessing mental health needs following disaster. *Psychiatric Annals* 34, 605–610.

Ritchie EC, Watson PJ and Friedman MJ (2006) *Interventions Following Mass Violence and Disaster Strategies for Mental Health Providers*. Guilford Press, New York.

Rosenberg RC (1994) The therapeutic alliance and the psychiatric emergency room crisis opportunity. *Psychiatric Annals* 24, 610–614.

Ruskin PE, Silver-Aylaiain M and Kling MA (2004) Treatment outcomes in depression: Comparison of remote treatment through telepsychiatry to in-person treatment. *American Journal of Psychiatry* 161(8), 1471–1476.

Sadock BJ and Sadock VA (2003) Child psychiatry: Assessment, examination, and psychological testing, in *Kaplan & Sadock's Synopsis of Psychiatry: Behavioral Sciences/Clinical Psychiatry*, 9th edn. Lippincott Williams & Wilkins, Philadelphia.

Schneider BJ (2006) Telepsychiatry and Walter Reed's virtual behavioral health clinic. Presentation at Psychiatry Grand Rounds University of Maryland School of Medicine, February.

Shea SC (1988) *Psychiatric Interviewing: The Art of Understanding*. WB Saunders Co., Philadelphia.

Ursano RJ, Fullerton CS and Norwood A (1995) Psychiatric dimensions if disaster: Patient care, community consultation, and preventive medicine. *Harvard Review of Psychiatry* 3, 196–209.

Ursano RJ, Fullerton CS and Norwood A (2003) *Terrorism and Disaster: Individual and Community Mental Health Interventions*. Cambridge University Press, Cambridge.

Welton RS (2007) The management of suicidality: Assessment and intervention. *Psychiatry* 4(5), 25–34.

Wise MG and Rundell JR (2005) *Clinical Manual of Psychosomatic Medicine: A Guide to Consultation-Liaison Psychiatry*. American Psychiatric Publishing, Inc., Washington, DC.

Yoshino A, Shigemura J, Kobayashi Y *et al.* (2001) Telepsychiatry: Assessment of televideo psychiatry interview reliability with present- and next-generation internet infrastructures. *Acta Psychiatrica Scandinavica* 104, 223–226.

Zur O (2012) TelePsychology or telementalhealth in the digital age: The future is here. *California Psychologist* 45, 13–15.

CHAPTER

6 Formulation

Allison Cowan, Randon Welton and Jerald Kay

The formulation must balance the simple and complex. If the formulation is too simple, it can overlook important knots that need to be unraveled. If a formulation is too complex, it only muddies efforts to think clearly about how to help. Our goal is a "just right" level of complexity.

Mardi J. Horowitz in *Formulations as a Basis for Planning Psychotherapy Treatment*

The objectives of the initial clinical interviews are to establish a safe therapeutic relationship and elicit critical information necessary for arriving at an accurate diagnosis and comprehensive treatment plan. An in-depth understanding of the patient is facilitated by the process of formulation. The formulation has been described as a hypothesis that demands refinement over time and considers the interplay of precipitants, causes, maintaining influences, and psychological factors as they relate to the mental life of the patient. These psychological factors include interpersonal and behavioral components as well as intrapsychic ones. Other authors have emphasized the importance of unconscious conflicts, deficits, and distortions from faulty intrapsychic structures, and internal object relations and their integration with "contemporary findings from the neurosciences" (Gabbard, 2010). This approach emphasizes the prominence of a gene and environment interaction. Neither biology nor experience is sufficient alone to arrive at a comprehensive appreciation of the patient's presentation. The formulation then is based on a biopsychosocial understanding of the patient with an appreciation of the deeper meanings of emotions and behaviors. Emphasizing those aspects operating outside the awareness of the patient prevents the biopsychosocial formulation from becoming a sterile recitation of the facts obtained during the interview. It will also help the formulation traverse the middle ground between, "… a descriptive diagnosis that refers to psychological and social issues, but is lacking in inference about psychological motivation to the extent that is does not provide an adequate guide for treatment" and a classic psychodynamic formulation that "…provides a refined and focused picture, but is seen as antiquated and not in keeping with the remarkable developments in neuroscience" (Summers, 2003).

Several arguments have historically been raised against the need for writing formulations, claiming they are archaic or strictly an academic exercise to be completed by residents without benefits "in the real world of clinical practice". The utility of the formulation is often improperly

The Psychiatric Interview: Evaluation and Diagnosis, First Edition. Allan Tasman, Jerald Kay and Robert J. Ursano.

confined to the ever-shrinking realm of long-term psychodynamic psychotherapy without an extension to modern treatment venues and practices (Perry *et al*., 2006). Some will argue that the formal formulation is unnecessary as long as the clinician diagnoses the patient according to the DSM-IV-TR. In this chapter, we will demonstrate the advantages of a more deeply informed formulation in the treatment of a variety of psychiatric patients. The formulation helps fill the gaps left by DSM-IV-TR axes and directs the treatment in a more individualized manner. "Case formulation can fill this gap between diagnosis and treatment and can be seen to lie at the intersection of etiology and description, theory and practice and science and art" (Sim *et al*., 2005). A biopsychosocial orientation can help guarantee that all pertinent areas of the patient's life are considered before the psychiatrist begins treatment (Clinical Vignette 1).

Clinical Vignette 1

Mr. G is a 54-year-old man who presents to the Emergency Department (ED) for "tightness" in his chest. He is accompanied by his teenage son. Mr. G reports pressure in his chest that is worse at rest. He appears anxious and diaphoretic. He tells the nurse, "You have to do something!"

Biological Contributions

For some patients, biological and medical issues may also present as psychological discomfort and/or pain. This is often the case for patients seen in consultation–liaison services where the impact of illness or the patient's response to illness is the driving force behind the consult request. Regardless of the setting, however, the biological or medical information gathered during the interview can deepen the understanding of the patient.

- *Family History of Mental Illness* – Most severe mental illnesses have a prominent genetic or heritable component. These issues require exploration to determine the patient's present and future vulnerability to life-altering conditions.
  - A 24-year-old woman presents for her second major depressive episode. She relates a prominent history of bipolar disorder in her family, with both her mother and brother suffering from the disease. This information will lead the psychiatrist to explore further for evidence of mania and hypomania in the patient's life and may influence the choice of medication to be prescribed.
- *Medical Illnesses* – The psychiatrist will want to explore medical conditions and note which have led to hospitalization or prolonged treatment. Previous treatments or recent changes in symptoms should be noted as well as serious medical conditions that run in the family. (Often exploration of this topic can provide an opportunity to inquire about the nature and helpfulness of previous doctor–patient relationships that may be a predictor of how well a patient can trust physicians, and therefore be a meaningful collaborator in care.) Special attention will be paid to illnesses that may induce or mimic psychiatric symptoms.
  - A 24-year-old woman presents for significant depressive symptoms. She has a personal and family history of thyroid condition. She has been taking thyroid replacement for years but has not had laboratory follow-up in the last year. Prior to beginning treatment for depression, the psychiatrist will want to check her thyroid functioning because hypothyroidism can lead to mood disturbance.

- *Medications* – The psychiatrist must ask about prescribed and over-the-counter medications since many medications and medication withdrawal can mimic psychiatric conditions. Patients may not consider herbal supplements as medications so these must be inquired about directly. When asking about medications, the clinician should further clarify if any of their medications have recently been started, stopped, or significantly changed.
  - A 32-year-old man comes in complaining of increased anxiety and panic attacks. He has recently experienced an exacerbation of asthma and was placed on "burst regimen" of steroids. The psychiatrist recognizes that the shortness of breath from the asthma as well as the steroids may be contributing to the patient's anxiety.
- *Substance Use* – Each patient should be queried about alcohol, illicit drugs, drugs of abuse, and tobacco. This includes current use, recent changes in use, and past use. Discovering that a patient has recently stopped using an illicit drug may help explain many symptoms. Helpful information can include amounts used, circumstances that lead to use, previous attempts to cut back use, and the impact use has had on his or her life.
- *Physical Condition* – Healthy living as characterized by adequate sleep, regular exercise, and a reasonable diet contribute significantly to mental wellness and resilience.
- *Neurovegetative Factors* – These form the basis for many DSM-IV-TR diagnoses. They include, for example, sleep, energy, appetite, and concentration.

Once biological factors have been identified, they will often be explored or addressed further. The 24-year-old woman with suspected thyroid disease will be referred for laboratory studies and additional workup. A patient with prominent sadness and neurovegetative symptoms may be a candidate for antidepressant medications. Sometimes, however, the treatment for these biological and medical problems will be social or psychological in nature, e.g., referral to AA for a recovering alcoholic, initiating cognitive-behavioral therapy in a patient with depression.

Clinical Vignette 1 (*continued*)

After reviewing the medical information and interviewing Mr. G, the psychiatric consultant discovers that Mr. G is suspected of having had a myocardial infarction (MI). His father and grandfather died in their early to mid 50s from heart attacks. Although his mother was always "nervous," there is no known family history of mental illness. Mr. G takes long-acting propranolol for his hypertension but he has been out of medication for several weeks. His busy schedule prevented him from going to the pharmacy. When the medical workup began to demonstrate that he did not have a heart attack, Mr. G became distraught and accused the physicians of making an error. That was when the ED physicians consulted psychiatry.

In this vignette, Mr. G has several biological factors that merit consideration. The most obvious need is to ensure that he is not having an MI. The psychiatrist serves in a special role in the medical community – dealing primarily with psychological complaints within a medical context. The psychiatrist's skill in eliciting information can often be beneficial for the entire medical team. Lastly, other key biological factors include Mr. G's family history of heart disease, anxiety, and his recently stopping his antihypertensive medication.

Social Factors

A comprehensive understanding of the patient's social situation provides a larger context for helping the psychiatrist to appreciate the patient as a product of the myriad of forces and situations they have experienced. It provides past academic, interpersonal, and occupational levels, thereby establishing a baseline of performance for the patient. Exploration of these issues may raise areas of interpersonal or intrapsychic vulnerabilities (e.g., the inability to maintain long-term relationships). The psychiatrist can also ascertain the patient's past efforts at adapting to life challenges and the availability of social support.

- *Cultural and Ethnic Heritage* – Only very rarely will a psychiatrist use this information to discover a "culturally bound syndrome", but for all patients, this information provides a view of identity and group membership. Moreover, the definition of mental illness and symptom description varies dramatically among different ethnocultural groups. The capacity to trust another in authority, the comfort about openness, the goals of treatment, the level of assertiveness, and gender issues are all highly relevant sociocultural factors. Patients from differing cultures may also embrace strong allegiance to family with less importance placed on individuality. Patients whose first language is not English mandate that close attention be paid to linguistic nuances.
    - A first-generation Asian-American college student was brought to the college mental health service by one of his professors who was concerned about the student's obvious depression and poor academic performance. She had asked the student repeatedly to seek help but he was reluctant to do so because of shame over his failure and stigma he perceived about psychiatric care.

Early Childhood Experiences

This can include the prosperity or poverty of the family as well as a broad overview of the quality of family relationships. Attachment experiences have enduring effects on personality development and lead to vulnerability or resilience to mental illness throughout the life cycle. The death or departure of parents or siblings can provide watershed moments in everyone's life. In addition, experiences in orphanages or foster care are often critical in early child development.

A 19-year-old man had attempted suicide after his wife of 6 months left him following a nonphysical argument. His description of his family of origin where "everyone yells at everyone else, but no one thinks of leaving" was very different than his wife's subdued childhood experiences, and pivotal in understanding the drama that led to this man's desperate action.

- *Abuse* – The presence of physical, sexual, or emotional abuse in childhood can forever change brain functioning and have significant repercussions in the ability to form satisfying relationships. It often makes potent contributions to self-worth and self-cohesiveness and needs to be asked about in a tactful yet direct manner. Although patients may not be willing to disclose this information at the first meeting, abuse of any form is frequently associated with psychiatric comorbidity and is important to identify as a topic that may be discussed in future treatment.
- *Academic History* – A patient's highest level of schooling as well as social experiences and grades in school can form a rough guide to their intelligence and

previous level of functioning. Participation in extracurricular activities and leadership positions often reflect reasonable sociability. How a student relates to teachers may reflect attitudes toward authority as well as toward learning environments.

- *Occupational Functioning* – This provides information into the patient's ability to function in a controlled setting and to compete with peers. The ability to tolerate changes and disappointments also provides helpful clues to adaptability. Current job performance and relationships with supervisors often portray patterns of enduring interpersonal difficulties and might be a factor in the patient's ability to continue treatment.
    - After a prolonged period of unemployment, a depressed 38-year-old man was recently hired as a mechanic at a small auto shop. The fact that he does not get paid for the time it takes to come to medical appointments may play a role in determining which types of treatment will be acceptable to him.

Relationships/Marital History

The ability to form and maintain relationships can be a key to understanding a patient's current circumstances. Obvious deficits in the ability to form relationships can itself be a focus of therapy and can be a reflection of the level of the availability of interpersonal support. Assessment of functioning within long-term committed relationships, friendships, marriage, and parent–child relationships is vital. The capacity for intimacy is critical to personality development. Inquiry should also be directed to the level of maturity and satisfaction in sexual intimacy as well.

- *Religious/Spiritual History* – For many patients, spiritual and/or religious beliefs are a key component in identity, daily functioning, and hope for the future. In addition, religious congregations can provide support and nurturance during difficult times. Equally, however, unpleasant or conflicted religious/spiritual experiences can be the cause of great ongoing distress.
    - A 37-year-old father of four has recently returned from a military deployment to a combat zone. His internist referred him to a psychiatrist for evaluation of depression. After a lifetime of religious involvement, the patient confides he is no longer sure if he can still believe in a god who would allow the "pointless destruction" of so many children during a "supposedly just war". Instituting antidepressant monotherapy clearly would not address some of the patient's intense doubts emanating from the recent active duty experiences.
- *Recent Stresses* – No matter how strong the genetic vulnerability, there is often an acute precipitant that initiates the mental illness or prompts the patient to seek help. The psychiatrist must reflect on the central question of "Why is the patient presenting at this time in need of treatment?" The psychiatrist should ask about recent changes in the individual's life circumstances or worsening of chronic situations. These can include recent psychological trauma and changes in the patient's legal, financial, academic, relational, or occupational problems.

Curiosity about the meaning of the symptoms to the patient is central in developing a formulation. It is also helpful to keep in mind that the presentation of illness or disturbance can not only reveal the focal or recent clinical issues but reflect on longstanding core or nuclear psychological issues as well.

Clinical Vignette 1 (*continued*)

Mr. G initially was focused on airing his grievances to the consultant about his "shabby" treatment by the ED staff, but he was cooperative. Mr. G was born into a white, working-class family with three siblings. "Things weren't always easy, but we had what we needed". He reported that his family moved around a lot due to his dad not being able to hold a job for long. His father was "strict, but he had to be with four kids. Mom wasn't much help". He reported that both his parents drank alcohol regularly, his mother more than his father, but defended them saying, "Times were different then. People weren't judged as much about it". He also denied abuse or neglect saying, "Sure we all got the belt, but it wasn't bad". Mr. G grew up in a nondenominational church but had stopped attending after he left home. He reported getting a scholarship to a state university from a local businessman. "I could have gotten into a better school if I had tried". He graduated with a degree in business and is currently in management at a medium-sized company. Mr. G reports that he has been under significant stress lately after he was passed over for a promotion. "I should have gotten it. That's why my wife left me. Twenty years together, and then she just leaves. She'll be back". Mr. G reported that his two younger children moved out with her, but their oldest son stayed with him. Mr. G reports that he drinks but that it is not a problem in his life. "I can hold my liquor".

Eliciting Mr. G's social history has uncovered significant new biological factors, including his use of alcohol and a potential family history of alcohol dependence. He has many recent stressors – his wife leaving with two of their children and his not getting a promotion. His childhood at this point remains mostly a mystery, but he had admitted that it "wasn't easy". He seems protective of his parents, so it is possible that he is censoring information that he feels might reflect poorly on them or has resentment toward them, which at this time he is unaware of.

Psychological Factors

Psychological factors encompass the breadth of the patient's internal mental world. Because they can be directly linked to specific psychotherapies, psychological factors are the most prone to being influenced by the theoretical orientation of the psychiatrist. The clinician who is a strong proponent of any one form of psychotherapy may preferentially attend to factors within that framework. Rather than having the theoretical orientation drive the formulation, however, it is preferable that the formulation determine the understanding of the patient and the selection of treatment modalities. By considering the full gamut of psychological factors, the psychiatrist will be prevented from prematurely narrowing the scope of his search. In the past, some have argued in favor of being true to one theoretical approach to the formulation. More prevalent today is the belief that drawing on a number of views enriches the clinician's understanding of the patient. Traditionally, these approaches have included efforts to understand a clinical presentation in terms of conflict or drive theory, ego psychology, object relations theory, self-psychology, cognitive behavioral theory, and more recently, attachment/intersubjective/relational dimensions. The last considers, for example, attachment styles, capacity for mentalization, and affect regulation (Table 6.1).

Table 6.1 Theoretical Approaches to Understanding a Patient

Drive theory
- Primary drives
- Defenses
- Origins of symptoms

Ego psychology
- Innate skills (conflict-free sphere)
- Early developmental influences
- Stressors
- Defenses/other adaptations
- Characterological development

Object relations
- Perception of self
- Perception of others
- Prevailing affective patterns

Self-psychology
- Grandiose pole
- Idealizable pole
- Innate skills and talents
- Self-regulatory capacity
- Capacity for joy/pleasure/humor

Attachment/intersubjective/relational dimensions
- Attachment style
- Capacity for mentalization/empathy
- Affective regulation

Cognitive behavioral theory (biased information-processing system)
- Maladaptive cognitive structures (schemas)
- Cognitive errors
- Negative automatic thoughts and images
- Compensatory strategies

Interpersonal theory (interpersonal non-psychoanalytic psychotherapy)
- Understanding the connection between life events and mood
- Selecting a problem area
  - Grief
  - Role transition
  - Role dispute
  - Interpersonal deficits

Source: For a more detailed explanation of psychoanalytically informed theoretical viewpoints, see Haggard PJ, Furman AC, Levy ST *et al.* (2008) Psychoanalytic theories, in *Psychiatry*, 3rd edn (eds Tasman A, Kay J, Lieberman JA *et al.*). John Wiley & Sons, Ltd, Chichester, pp. 464–482.

- *Coping Strategies* – The psychiatrist will need to assess the patient's ability to cope with change and with stress. Much of this will align with an assessment of what has traditionally been called ego strength. Considerations can include the following:
    - How does the patient deal with adversity?
    - Can the patient adapt to sudden change?
    - How does the patient deal with strong emotions?
    - Can the patient consistently pursue healthy goals?
    - Psychological defenses should also be assessed, and especially those defense mechanisms that are used in dealing with emotional distress should be noted.
        - Mature defenses include humor, suppression, and altruism.
        - Intermediate defenses include undoing, intellectualization, rationalization, or isolation of affect.
        - Less mature strategies include denial, repression, acting out, projection, or splitting.

Table 6.2 provides a summary of some common defense mechanisms.

- Is the patient able to imagine a point of view different from their own (mentalization)? What is the capacity for empathy?
- What is the patient's capacity for psychological mindedness?

Table 6.2 Some Common Defense Mechanisms (Kay and Kay, 2008)*

Denial	Refusal to appreciate information about oneself or others
Projection	Attribution to others of one's own unacceptable thoughts or feelings
Projective identification	Attribution of unacceptable personality characteristics to another followed by an attempt to develop a relationship based on those characteristics
Regression	A partial return to earlier levels of adaptation to avoid conflict
Splitting	Experiencing of others as being all good or all bad, i.e., idealization or devaluation and acting upon it
Conversion	Transformation of unacceptable wishes or thoughts into body sensations
Reaction formation	Transformation of an unwanted thought or feeling into its opposite
Isolation	Divorcing a feeling from its unpleasant idea
Rationalization	Using seemingly logical explanations to make untenable feelings or thoughts more acceptable
Displacement	Redirection of unpleasant feelings or thoughts onto another object
Dissociation	Splitting off thought or feeling from its original source
Sublimation	A mature mechanism whereby unacceptable thoughts and feelings are channeled into socially acceptable ones

*All defense mechanisms are involuntary and unconscious and are arranged approximately from immature to more mature defenses.

Morality/Conscientiousness

Whether it is conceptualized as superego strength, an abiding schema, or core beliefs, the psychiatrist should explore the capacity for maintaining appropriate societal norms. Is his or her sense of morality somewhat loose or overly rigid? Does honesty and conscientiousness characterize interactions with others?

- *Cognitions* – Does the patient have characteristic thought patterns, which either aid or detract from their health and functioning? Unhealthy thought patterns could include extreme pessimism, self-deprecation, or irrational condemnation of their own actions. As the patient describes the events of their life, the psychiatrist will listen for themes that persist no matter what topic is being discussed.
  - A 21-year-old college student is being seen on a medical unit. He was admitted for gastritis and expresses significant anxiety and depression. The gastritis seems to be secondary to frequent caffeine and tobacco use. He feels that he is inadequate and will fail his classes. This leads him to study for 6–7 hours per day, requiring the regular use of stimulants. He complains that even this is unhelpful, as his grades have been falling to a B average. A discussion with the psychiatrist demonstrates a tendency to believe that he is about to experience devastating losses. This applies to his grades and his relationships with family and his girlfriend.
- *Behaviors* – The clinician must ascertain recent changes in behaviors. Have hobbies, other activities, or interests become less gratifying? The psychiatrist should inquire about unhealthy, repetitive, and/or self-destructive behavior. Although the underlying cause of these behavioral shifts may not be evident initially, their exploration and management may become a major thrust of therapy. Positive changes in behavior should also be noted.
- *Relationships* – The clinical significance of both the number and quality of the patient's relationships has been discussed previously. In this section, however, the psychiatrist is looking in more depth at characterizing current interpersonal relationships. Can the patient initiate and maintain stable, rewarding relationships? Is there a pattern of engaging in unhealthy or distressing relationships? If so, what role is usually played? Are there unrealistic expectations of others with whom they have significant relationships? What can be said about this patient's capacity for intimacy? Would he characterize his sexual relationships as gratifying and mature?
  - A 25-year-old woman presents with symptoms of anxiety and mood lability following her somewhat impetuous resignation at work. She reported that other women always hate her because they are jealous of her. She disclosed that her father always preferred her, but that her mother "ran him off". She has found it difficult to stay in treatment with female therapists in the past. Examining her long-standing conflicts with women would undoubtedly be helpful in understanding her mood and anxiety symptoms.

Given the ubiquity of interpersonal problems in those seeking or needing help, the formulation process is invaluable in teasing out the contributing factors to poorly relating to others.

Self-Esteem

As noted earlier, the assessment of a patient's identity and the nature and stability of self-esteem is often critical. In addition to expressions about self-worth and competence, the ability to self-soothe at times of distress in a nondestructive manner provides insight into a patient's ability to pursue desires and ambitions.

- *Meaning and Significance* – Throughout the interview, the psychiatrist can listen for experiences, beliefs, or activities that bring significance and purpose into a patient's life. Does helping others, for example, provide such meaningful experiences?

Clinical Vignette 1 (*continued*)

"That idiot doctor down in the ER didn't even know what he was talking about". The psychiatrist continues the interview by asking what Mr. G thought was happening with his health. Mr. G reported that the doctor probably missed something important because he hadn't listened as closely as he should have. "Nobody listens to me – not my boss, not my wife, and not my two kids that she turned against me". Mr. G reported that he felt the interviewer really listened to him and was immensely helpful. He reported that his chest was still a little tight but that he was feeling better.

Coping Strategies – Mr. G appears to be relying on denial as a main coping strategy in his interview. This is demonstrated by his being unable to accept the results of his medical tests and his not believing his wife has permanently left him. In times of great stress like medical illness and extreme marital discord, an individual's defenses are especially challenged. Mr. G also struggles with dealing with strong emotions as his outburst in the ED shows. Although there is insufficient evidence at this point, it might be useful to determine if Mr. G might also be using alcohol to modulate his feelings.

Morality/Conscientiousness – Mr. G reports that it isn't fair that other people get to do whatever they want at work, but when he does it, his boss writes him up. This helped the examiner understand that Mr. G might have difficulties understanding the subtleties of right and wrong and may think that the rules do not apply to him. This would constitute evidence for a sense of entitlement and grandiosity.

Cognitions – Mr. G appears to believe that no one listens to him. While this may be mostly true, it also may represent, as conceptualized from a cognitive behavioral therapy orientation, a deep-seated negative, automatic schema.

Relationships – Mr. G has recently had three very important relationships change dramatically, namely, those with his wife and two children. From an object relations viewpoint, the psychiatrist should consider what kind of internal representations of others populate his patient's inner world. Does he believe that people are more likely than not to use him for their own needs? Does he think that people dismiss him without giving him his due like his wife and the ED physician? Is he able to integrate good and bad characteristics of one person without it radically changing his view of them?

- *Relating to the Interviewer* – The patient's attitude toward the interviewer is a rich source of information. It can often be used to extrapolate patterns to the other relationships in the patient's life. These attitudes are commonly outside of the patient's awareness and illustrate a central tenant of psychodynamic theory called transference. Additionally, the interviewer's feelings toward the patient (countertransference) can be informative, especially if the interviewer's reactions are out of the range they normally experience. Countertransference is ubiquitous and affords the psychiatrist an additional vehicle for assessment and formulation. Indeed, many formulation formats include formal observation and recording of transference and countertransference because both concepts offer the opportunity to anticipate major themes and challenges in psychotherapy.

As the psychiatrist understands the internal experiences of the patient, treatment options can be developed which match the patient's strengths and deficits. These persisting psychological patterns along with the competence of the therapist and the patient's wishes will help determine which therapeutic approach is most likely to be successful.

- Mr. G reports that his wife was "great" until she became active in a community group, which led to arguments about how she spent her time. He reported, "She became a totally different person. She got selfish and rude". He is also unable or unwilling to endorse negative qualities about his parents.

Although it is unlikely that Mr. G's wife had a sudden change in personality, it is a possibility. More likely, however, is that Mr. G began to feel neglected, a common theme throughout his life. If this were approached from an interpersonal psychotherapy perspective, Mr. G's role dispute/change would be important to work through. Examining attachment experiences in his childhood may better inform the psychiatrist as to how Mr. G attaches to others as an adult (easily, in a conflicted manner, or not at all).

Self-Esteem – Mr. G initially appears demanding and entitled in the ED. However, this may be a reflection of his anxiety. Given his significant recent losses both at work and home, Mr. G's self-esteem is likely at a low point. Given his reliance on somatization to cope with this adversity, it is unlikely that he is able to soothe himself in an adaptive fashion.

Meaning and Significance – Striking in its absence is what makes Mr. G's life meaningful. Sometimes in interviews how a person finds meaning and significance is clear: parenthood, religious or political affiliation, or through work. However, in some cases, it is a mystery even to the patient. Helping the patient explore this issue can, in itself, be therapeutic.

Relating to the Interviewer – Mr. G seems to have taken to the interviewer in the vignette. This may be the result of the interviewer's benign curiosity and/or a sense of his desperation being finally acknowledged. It, also, may be reenacting an earlier relationship with a predetermined script, e.g., initially idealizing the interviewer, then after a real or perceived therapeutic misstep devaluing them as was the case with the ED staff.

Summary

The formulation allows the psychiatrist to develop an explanatory hypothesis about a patient's current psychological difficulties by bringing together pertinent factors from the entirety of the patient's life and experiences. By considering these different areas, the psychiatrist can develop a broader and more in-depth understanding of the patient, which examines all sectors of personality and development as well as both previous and current levels of psychosocial functioning and capacity for adaptation. Not every patient will have pertinent information in every category, but the psychiatrist should consider each of these categories seriously. This understanding should then be essential in the development of a comprehensive treatment plan, with the psychiatrist focused on the areas where change is likely, or alternately, helping the patient "learn to accept unalterable conditions when necessary" (Horowitz, 1997). The formulation is invaluable in the identification and the meaning of problematic issues within a biopsychosocial context.

References

Gabbard G (2010) *Long-Term Psychodynamic Psychotherapy*. American Psychiatric Publishing Inc., Washington, DC.

Horowitz MJ (1997) *Formulations as a Basis for Planning Psychotherapy Treatment*. American Psychiatric Publishing Inc., Washington, DC.

Kay J and Kay RL (2008) Individual psychoanalytic psychotherapy, in *Psychiatry* (eds Tasman A, Kay J, Lieberman JA *et al.*), 3rd edn. John Wiley & Sons, Ltd, Chichester, pp. 1851–1874.

Perry S, Cooper AM and Michels R (2006) The psychodynamic formulation: Its purpose, structure, and clinical application. *Focus* 4, 297–305.

Sim K, Gwee KP and Bateman A (2005) Case formulation in psychotherapy: Revitalizing its usefulness as a clinical tool. *Academic Psychiatry* 29, 289–292.

Summers RF (2003) The psychodynamic formulation updated. *American Journal of Psychotherapy* 57, 39–51.

CHAPTER

7 Clinical Evaluation and Treatment Planning: A Multimodal Approach

The complete psychiatric evaluation consists of the psychiatric interview; physical examination, including neurological assessment; laboratory testing; and, as appropriate, neuropsychological testing, structured interviews, and brain imaging. The results of the evaluation are used to assess risk, reach diagnoses, and complete initial and comprehensive treatment plans. The length, detail, and order of the evaluation need to be modified when it is conducted in different settings. The clinician needs to assess the goals of the interview, the patient's tolerance for questioning, and the time available. Table 7.1 shows the variation of the psychiatric evaluation with the type of setting.

Psychiatric Interview

The psychiatric interview (Table 7.2) is the cornerstone of clinical evaluation in psychiatry. It is essential for establishing rapport with the patient, initiating the therapeutic alliance, eliciting the psychiatric history, and performing the Mental Status Examination (MSE). When conducted skillfully, the interview may appear to be a relaxed and casual conversation. However, it is actually an extremely precise diagnostic tool composed of specific elements: the identifying information, the chief complaint, the history of present illness, the past psychiatric history, the personal history, the family history, the medical history, the substance use history, and the MSE.

Before beginning, the psychiatrist should introduce himself or herself, explain the purpose of the interview, and make the patient as comfortable as possible. The interview gives the most accurate information when the psychiatrist and patient speak in a language in which they are both fluent. When this is not possible, a translator should be used, preferably one with mental health training or experience. Even then, some of the subtleties of the patient's communications are lost.

The Psychiatric Interview: Evaluation and Diagnosis, First Edition. Allan Tasman, Jerald Kay and Robert J. Ursano.

This chapter is based on Chapter 30 (Francine Cournos, David A. Lowenthal, Deborah L. Cabaniss) of *Psychiatry*, 3rd Edition.

Table 7.1 Psychiatric Evaluation and Treatment Planning

Setting	Psychiatric Interview and Mental Status Examination (MSE)	Physical or Neurological Examination, Laboratory Assessments, Brain Imaging	Treatment Planning
Emergency room	Most often lengthy and extensive, except as limited by patient's ability or willingness to communicate.	Physical examination is often performed; other tests and examinations are ordered as indicated.	Primary focus is on disposition.
Psychiatric inpatient unit	Extensive, but complete information may be obtained in a series of interviews over time.	Physical and neurological examinations and laboratory tests are always performed; other tests and examinations are ordered as indicated.	Comprehensive and formal plans are developed.
Consultation liaison service	Depth of interview is highly variable depending on reasons for referral and patient's medical condition; an attempt is made to obtain a complete MSE.	Most medical information is obtained from the chart; psychiatric consultant may request further assessment.	Recommendations focus on reasons for referral and are made to the primary treatment team.
Outpatient office or clinic	Urgency of situation is assessed; in nonurgent situations, the initial interview usually focuses on the chief complaint and MSE.	Medical information is obtained as needed, usually by referral to a general practitioner or specialist.	Planning may be formal or informal, depending on applicable regulatory and reimbursement requirements.
Third-party interviews (e.g., for court, disability determinations)	Interview addresses the reason for referral and may be narrowly focused but contains a complete MSE.	Assessments are ordered according to the purpose of the interview.	Not usually relevant except for recommendations pertaining to the purpose of the interview.

Table 7.2	Psychiatric Interview
Greeting Identifying information Chief complaint History of present illness Past psychiatric history Personal history Family history Medical history Substance use history Mental status examination	

Identifying Information

Most interviewers find it helpful to begin with a few questions designed to identify the patient in a general way. Asking the patient's name, age, address, marital status, and occupation provides a quick general picture and begins the interview with emotionally neutral material. If the interviewer chooses to begin in this way, it is important to complete this section rapidly and then give the patient a chance to respond to open-ended questions. This allows the interviewer to gain a more accurate sense of the patient's spontaneous speech patterns, thought processes, and thought content. If the patient becomes too disorganized in response to this change, the psychiatrist can revert to more focused questions to structure and organize the interview. If it is possible, within the context of the interview, other pieces of identifying information, such as the patient's ethnic group and religious affiliation, should be obtained.

Chief Complaint

At the start, the interviewer wants to ascertain exactly why the patient is seeking psychiatric help at this time. The interviewer may begin with a fairly general question, such as "What brings you to treatment at this time?" The patient may have a long history of psychiatric illness, but the chief complaint refers only to the acute problem that necessitates the current intervention. The interviewer should try to help the patient distinguish the chief complaint from any chronic problems, as in the following example:

Interviewer: Can you tell me what brings you to see a psychiatrist at this time?
Patient: Well, I have had schizophrenia for 25 years.
Interviewer: I see. But my guess is that something happened recently that has prompted you to come in today, rather than several months ago.
Patient: Oh, yes. Yesterday my wife kicked me out of the house. I'm homeless.

Here the patient's chief complaint is homelessness; the schizophrenia is part of his psychiatric history. Although a psychotic patient may offer a chief complaint that seems incoherent or unrealistic, it is important to collect the chief complaint in the patient's words and later look to other sources of information for additional history. Similarly, in response to the question, "What brings you to seek psychotherapy at this time?" a patient may begin to answer by detailing his or her childhood, but the interviewer should help the patient to focus on current issues that precipitated the consultation. Some patients may not be able to cite a chief complaint: "My wife sent me" or "There's no problem. I don't know why the police picked me up". Even these answers give the interviewer information about the patient's current situation, which can be elaborated on by asking the patient for more details.

History of Present Illness

The interviewer should clarify the nature of the present illness. The present illness begins with the onset of signs and symptoms that characterize the current episode of illness. For example, the present illness of a manic patient with chronic bipolar disorder who was asymptomatic for the past 3 years would begin with the onset of the current episode of mania. The interviewer determines the duration of the present illness, as well as precipitating factors such as psychosocial stressors, substance use, discontinuing medication, and medical illnesses. The patient should be allowed to tell the story, and the clinician should follow up with specific diagnostic questions.

Past Psychiatric History

The interviewer should ask for information regarding any previous episodes of psychiatric illness or treatment, including hospitalization, medications, outpatient therapy, substance use treatment, self-help groups, and consultation with culture-specific healers such as shamans. The duration and effectiveness of treatment should be ascertained, as well as the patient's general experience of his or her psychiatric treatment to date.

Personal History

Within the constraints of the interviewer's time and the patient's tolerance for further questioning, the clinician should inquire about the patient's upbringing, educational and vocational history, interpersonal relations, and current social situation. It is important to inquire about the patient's sexual history and to ask about risk factors for human immunodeficiency virus (HIV) infection, such as a history of multiple partners, unprotected vaginal and anal intercourse, and intravenous drug use. This information is relevant not only for the assessment and diagnosis of the present illness but also for treatment planning (Table 7.3).

Table 7.3 Personal History

Prenatal history
Wanted vs. unwanted pregnancy
History of maternal malnutrition or maternal drug use (including prescription drugs)
Circumstances of birth (vaginal delivery vs. cesarean section)
History of birth trauma
Birth order
Early childhood (0–3 years)
Temperament
Major milestones, including speech and motor development
History of toilet training
Early feeding history, including breast-feeding
Early behavioral problems (e.g., nightmares and night terrors, enuresis and encopresis, aggressive behavior)
Early relationships with parents and siblings
History of significant early illnesses or hospitalizations
History of early separations from caregivers
Middle childhood – latency (3–11 years)
Early school history, including any evidence of cognitive impairment
Relationships with siblings and peers
Early personality development
History of behavioral problems (e.g., separation anxiety, school phobia, aggressive behavior)
Adolescence (12–18 years)
Psychosexual development, including experience of puberty and menarche, masturbatory history, and early sexual behavior
Later school history
Later personality development
History of behavioral or emotional problems (e.g., substance abuse, eating disorders)
Adulthood
Marital history or history of relationships with significant others
History of child-rearing
Sexual history
Occupational and educational history
Religious history
Current living situation

Family History

The interviewer should ask the patient specifically about any relatives with a history of psychiatric illness, psychiatric treatment, suicide attempts, or substance use. This information is important for diagnosis as well as for treatment planning. For example, a patient who presents with a first episode of acute psychosis may have any one of a number of disorders, but a family history of affective disorders may lead the interviewer to suspect a diagnosis of bipolar disorder or major depression with psychotic features rather than schizophrenia.

Medical History

A careful review of a patient's medical history is an important part of the psychiatric interview because medical conditions can dramatically affect psychiatric status. Many medical disorders such as endocrinological conditions (thyroid disease, pheochromocytomas, pituitary adenomas), neurological disorders (Parkinson's disease, central nervous system neoplasms, Wilson's disease, stroke syndromes, head trauma), and infectious diseases (HIV infection, meningitis, sepsis) can have manifestations that include psychiatric symptoms . A review of all of the patient's medications, including over-the-counter preparations and alternative remedies, is important because many of these substances can produce or exacerbate psychiatric symptoms.

Substance Use History

The interviewer should inquire about which substances are used, under what circumstances, and the quantity, variety, and duration of use (Table 7.4). A question such as "Do

Table 7.4 Substance Use History
Survey of drugs that have been used include:
Alcohol
Opioids (heroin, methadone, analgesics)
Stimulants (cocaine, crack, amphetamines, ecstasy)
Depressants (benzodiazepines, barbiturates)
Hallucinogens (cannabis, lysergic acid diethylamide [LSD], mescaline)
Phencyclidine
Nicotine
Caffeine
Over-the-counter preparations
Pattern of usage
Age of first use
Period of heaviest use
Pattern or frequency of current use
Route of administration (injected, intranasal, inhaled, oral)
Periods of sobriety
Symptoms of tolerance or dependence
Medical history, including HIV status and other substance use-related disorders; note ongoing substance use despite knowledge that it could worsen medical conditions
History of treatment for substance use
Legal history; note relationship to drug use

Table 7.5 Human Immunodeficiency Virus Risk Factors

Parenteral
Use of shared needles or drug works in the course of drug injection or amateur tattooing
Receipt of blood, blood products, or organ transplant in the USA between 1978 and 1985
Maternal–fetal transmission (pediatric cases)
Occupational exposure among health-care workers and laboratory technicians through needle-stick injuries and other significant exposures (uncommon)
Unsafe sexual activity
Most common for men: unprotected anal intercourse with other men; unprotected vaginal or anal intercourse with women who are known to be HIV-positive, engage in prostitution, or are injection drug users or sexual partners of injection drug users; multiple heterosexual partners
Most common for women: unprotected anal or vaginal intercourse with men who are known to be HIV-positive, are injection drug users, are the sexual partners of injection drug users, are bisexual, or were treated for hemophilia or coagulation disorder when blood products were contaminated; multiple heterosexual partners
Cofactors
Compromise of the skin or mucous membranes, especially through the presence of sexually transmitted diseases, which increases the likelihood of transmission on exposure to HIV-infected body fluids
Use of noninjection drugs, especially alcohol and crack cocaine, through association with high-risk sexual activity
Environmental context
Risk behavior while living or traveling in geographic areas with high rates of HIV infection, through increased likelihood of exposure to HIV-infected body fluids

you drink alcohol?" is likely to be answered with a quick "No". A better question, such as "How much alcohol do you drink?", communicates to the patient that the clinician is not making a value judgment and is more likely to elicit an accurate answer (Table 7.5).

Mental Status Examination

The MSE is a structured way to assess a patient's mental state at a given time. Unlike the parts of the interview that focus on the history, the MSE provides a descriptive snapshot of the patient at the interview. Much of the information needed for the evaluation of appearance, behavior, and speech is gathered without specific questioning during the course of the interview. Bearing in mind the outline of the MSE (Table 7.6) ensures that the interview is comprehensive.

Table 7.6 Mental Status Examination

I. Appearance
II. Behavior (includes attitude toward the interviewer)
III. Speech
IV. Mood and affect
V. Thought
 A. Thought process
 B. Thought content
VI. Perception
 A. Hallucinations
  1. Auditory
  2. Visual
  3. Other (somatic, gustatory, tactile)
 B. Illusions
VII. Cognition
 A. Level of awareness
 B. Level of alertness
 C. Orientation
  1. Person
  2. Place
  3. Time
 D. Memory
  1. Immediate
  2. Short term
  3. Long term
 E. Attention (digit span)
 F. Calculations
 G. Fund of knowledge
 H. Abstractions
  1. Similarities
  2. Proverbs
 I. Insight
 J. Judgment

Appearance

The interviewer should note the patient's general appearance, including grooming, level of hygiene, and attire.

Behavior

This includes the patient's level of cooperativeness with the interview, motor excitement or retardation, abnormal movements (e.g., tardive dyskinesia, tremors), and maintenance of eye contact with the interviewer.

Speech

The psychiatrist should carefully assess the patient's speech for rate, fluency, clarity, and softness or loudness. The interviewer may want to question the patient directly about striking or symptomatic aspects of his or her speech such as its speed or speech impediments.

Mood and Affect

The interviewer should note the patient's mood and affect. This may be evident from the way in which the patient answers other questions and tells the history, but specific questions are often indicated. The patient's mood is a pervasive affective state, and it is often helpful simply to ask, "What has your mood been like lately?" or "How would you describe your mood?" In contrast, affect is the way in which one modulates and conveys one's feeling state from moment to moment. The clinician judges the congruity between the material the patient is presenting and the accompanying affect, that is, sadness when discussing the death of a loved one or happiness when describing a child's accomplishments. This reveals whether the affect is labile (shifts too rapidly) and whether it is appropriate to the content of the material .

Thought

The clinician assesses the patient's thought process and content. Thought process is the form of the patient's thoughts – are they organized and goal directed or are they tangential, circumstantial, or loosely associated? If the patient's thought processes are difficult to understand, the clinician can indicate his or her difficulty in following what is being said and then assess the patient's response to this intervention. Some patients – such as patients with stroke who have nonfluent aphasias – may appear to have disorganized speech but are aware that they are not making sense, whereas those with fluent aphasias, psychosis, and delirium are not necessarily aware of their impairment. The psychiatrist should ask specifically about the patient's thought content, including delusions (grandiose, persecutory, somatic), hallucinations (auditory, visual, tactile, and olfactory), obsessions, phobias, and suicidal and homicidal ideation. Although these questions should be asked with tact and empathy, they should always be asked. Patients are generally relieved that the interviewer has broached the subject of suicide, and simply asking the question does not give patients ideas they have not had before.

Cognition

Every psychiatric interview should include some assessment of the patient's cognitive functioning. This includes the patient's level of awareness, alertness, and orientation (to person, place, and time). If there is a question about the patient's memory, formal memory testing may be done to assess short-term, intermediate, and long-term memory. A patient who can answer questions for 30 minutes is clearly attentive, but any doubts about the patient's attentiveness should prompt a formal assessment, for example, asking the patient to recite a series of digits forward and backward. Before assessing the patient's calculations and fund of knowledge, it is important to ascertain the patient's level of education. Formal assessment of the patient's ability to abstract may be unnecessary for a patient who has used abstract constructions throughout the interview, but the interviewer may want to ask formally for interpretations of similes and proverbs. It is often helpful to begin with simple constructions, for example, asking the patient the meaning of such phrases as "He has a warm heart" or "Save your money for a rainy day". Patients whose native language is not English may have difficulty in this area, which does not reflect a lack of ability to abstract.

The interviewer should gain a full understanding of the patient's insight into the illness by asking why, in the patient's opinion, he or she is currently in need of psychiatric care and what has caused problems. Finally, the interviewer should learn about the patient's judgment. This is best assessed in terms of the circumstances of the patient's life, for example, asking a mother how she would deal with a situation in which she had to leave her children to go to the store or asking a chronically ill person what he does when he sees that he is running out of medicine.

The interviewer may want to use the Mini-Mental State Examination (Mini-MSE) to quantify the degree of cognitive impairment of a patient with obvious cognitive

Maximum Score	Score	
		ORIENTATION
5	( )	What is the (year) (season) (date) (day) (month)?
5	( )	Where are we: (state) (county) (town) (hospital) (floor)?
		REGISTRATION
3	( )	Name 3 objects: 1 second to say each. Then ask the patient all 3 after you have said them. Give 1 point for each correct answer. Then repeat them until he learns all 3. Count trials and record. Trials
		ATTENTION AND CALCULATION
5	( )	Serial 7's. 1 point for each correct. Stop after 5 answers. Alternatively spell "world" backwards.
		RECALL
3	( )	Ask for the 3 objects repeated above. Give 1 point for each correct.
		LANGUAGE
9	( )	Name a pencil, and a watch (2 points) Repeat the following "No ifs, ands or buts." (1 point) Follow a 3-stage command: "Take a paper in your right hand, fold it in half, and put it on the floor" (3 points) Ready and obey the following: CLOSE YOUR EYES (1 point) Write a sentence (1 point) Copy design (1 point)
________		Total score ASSESS level of consciousness along a continuum ________ Alert Drowsy Stupor Coma

Figure 7.1 *Mini-mental state examination* (*Source*: Folstein MF, Folstein SE and McHugh PR (1975) "Mini-mental state": A practical method for grading the cognitive state of patients for the clinician. *Journal of Psychiatric Research* 12, 189–198 (reprinted with permission from Elsevier Science, Pergamon Imprint, Oxford)).

abnormalities. This can be useful as an initial diagnostic tool, as well as a means of assessing changes in cognitive function over time. The Mini-MSE is outlined in Figure 7.1.

Physical Examination

The physical examination is an important part of the comprehensive psychiatric evaluation. Many patients who present with psychiatric symptoms may have underlying medical problems that are causing or exacerbating the presenting symptoms. For example, an agitated, delirious patient may be septic or a patient being treated for an autoimmune disorder who develops new onset paranoia may have a steroid-induced psychosis. Assessing the patient's physical capacity to tolerate certain psychiatric medications, such as tricyclic antidepressants or lithium, is also important. Finally, many patients who present to a psychiatrist have had inadequate medical care and should be routinely examined to assess their general level of physical health. This is especially true for patients with chronic mental illness or substance abuse. In some settings, such as emergency rooms and inpatient wards, the psychiatrist may want to perform the physical examination; in others, it may be more appropriate to refer the patient to a general practitioner for this purpose. Genital, rectal, and breast examinations can usually be included even for anxious and paranoid patients, but when they must be postponed, care should be taken to complete them at a later time. A same-sex chaperone is necessary for the security of both the patient and the examiner.

Certain aspects of the information obtained in the psychiatric interview should alert the psychiatrist to the need for a physical examination. Any indication (Table 7.7) from the history that the psychiatric symptoms followed physical trauma, infection, medical illness, or drug ingestion should prompt a full physical examination. Similarly, the acute onset of psychiatric symptoms in a previously psychiatrically healthy individual, as well as symptoms arising at an unusual age, should raise questions about potential medical causes (Table 7.8).

Physical examination may also be warranted during treatment with medication if physical symptoms arise.

Table 7.7 Indications for Physical Examination
History of medical illness
Current symptoms of medical illness, particularly fever, neurological symptoms, or cardiovascular abnormalities
Evidence while taking history of altered mental status or cognitive impairment
History or physical evidence of trauma, particularly head trauma
Rapid onset of symptoms
New onset of psychosis, depression, mania, panic attacks
New onset of visual, tactile, or olfactory hallucinations
New onset psychiatric symptoms after age 40
Family history of physical illness that could cause psychiatric illness

Table 7.8 Physical Illnesses That May Present with Psychiatric Symptoms

Neurological	Metabolic
Amyotrophic lateral sclerosis	Acute intermittent porphyria
Epilepsy – particularly partial complex seizures (e.g., temporal lobe epilepsy)	Electrolyte imbalance
Huntington's disease	Hepatic encephalopathy
Multi-infarct dementia	Hepatolenticular degeneration (Wilson's disease)
Normal-pressure hydrocephalus	Hypoxemia
Parkinson's disease	Uremic encephalopathy
Pick's disease	**Nutritional**
Stroke syndromes (cerebrovascular disease)	Vitamin B_{12} deficiency
Rheumatological (autoimmune)	Central pontine myelinolysis
Systemic lupus erythematosus	Folate deficiency (megaloblastic anemia)
Temporal arteritis	General malnutrition
Infectious	Nicotinic acid deficiency (pellagra)
Acquired immunodeficiency syndrome	Thiamine deficiency (Wernicke–Korsakoff syndrome)
Brain abscess	Infectious
Encephalitis	**Traumatic, particularly head**
General infection (e.g., urinary tract)	**Trauma toxic**
Meningitis	Environmental toxins
Syphilis, particularly neurosyphilis	Intoxication with alcohol or other drugs
Tuberculosis	**Neoplastic**
Viral hepatitis	Carcinoma (general)
Endocrine	Central nervous system tumors (primary or metastatic)
Adrenal hyperplasia (Cushing's syndrome)	Endocrine tumors
Diabetes mellitus	Pancreatic carcinoma
Hypo- or hyperparathyroidism	
Hypo- or hyperthyroidism	
Hypothalamic dysfunction	
Panhypopituitarism	
Pheochromocytoma	

Neurological Examination

With every patient, the psychiatrist should consider a thorough neurological examination, especially for hospitalized patients. Patients who have a history of neurological disturbances, such as strokes, seizure disorders, central nervous system neoplasms, dementias, and movement disorders, should be carefully evaluated, perhaps by a neurologist. The neurological examination should be particularly designed to rule out any lateralizing neurological signs that would point toward the presence of a focal lesion.

Psychological and Neuropsychological Testing

Psychological and neuropsychological tests are standard instruments used to measure specific aspects of mental functioning. They are usually administered by psychologists or other professionals who have been trained in their use and interpretation. In most cases, several tests, often referred to as a battery, are performed together. These test results must then be interpreted in the context of the broad clinical picture of the patient.

Structured Clinical Instruments and Rating Scales

Structured instruments and rating scales have been developed for clinical and for research purposes. They allow clinicians to track symptoms and investigators to compare findings in different studies by ensuring that similar data and criteria have been used to establish diagnoses and to measure the presence and severity of psychiatric symptoms and their response to treatment. Many types of mental health professionals and, in some cases, nonclinicians can be trained to administer these rating scales.

Although most practicing clinicians do not commonly use structured instruments to assess or follow up patients, a small number of rating scales have come to be used routinely in clinical practice. For example, the PHQ-9 for depression, the PCL-17 for PTSD, and the Abnormal Involuntary Movement Scale (Figure 7.2) to monitor patients receiving antipsychotic medication for the presence of tardive dyskinesia, and the Global Assessment of Functioning Scale.

Laboratory Assessments

A variety of laboratory tests can aid in the clinical evaluation of the psychiatric patient (Table 7.9) (Council on Scientific Affairs, 1987; Gold and Dackis, 1986).

Neurophysiologic Assessment

A variety of techniques are now available that can provide more direct assessments of brain function in psychiatric patients. These include not only neuroimaging techniques (positron emission tomography (PET) scans and functional magnetic resonance imaging (MRI)), but also electrophysiologic measures, such as the electroencephalogram (EEG) and evoked or event-related potentials (ERPs). Electrophysiologic measures have the advantage of being economical and noninvasive, and allow continuous monitoring of brain electrical activity with a temporal resolution that surpasses that of neuroimaging measures. The EEG has traditionally been used in psychiatry to screen for brain disorders. In a conventional clinical EEG, a highly trained reader uses visual inspection of brain waves recorded from scalp electrodes. The presence of epileptiform discharges, spikes, or generalized slowing of brain electrical activity is associated with known central

INSTRUCTIONS: Complete Examination Procedure before making ratings.
MOVEMENT RATINGS: Rate highest severity observed.
Rate movements that occur upon activation one *less* than those observed spontaneously.

Code: 0 = None
1 = Minimal, may be extreme normal
2 = Mild
3 = Moderate
4 = Severe

		(Circle One)				
FACIAL AND ORAL MOVEMENTS:	1. Muscles of facial expression e.g., movements of forehead, eyebrows, periorbital area, cheeks; include, frowning, blinking, smiling, grimacing	0	1	2	3	4
	2. Lips and perioral area e.g., puckering, pouting, smacking	0	1	2	3	4
	3. Jaw e.g., biting, clenching, chewing, mouth opening, lateral movement	0	1	2	3	4
	4. Tongue Rate only increase in movement both in and out of mouth, NOT inability to sustain movement	0	1	2	3	4
EXTREMITY MOVEMENTS:	5. Upper *(arms, wrists, hands, fingers)* include choreic movements (i.e., rapid, objectively purposeless, irregular, spontaneous), athetoid movements (i.e., slow, irregular, complex, serpentine) Do NOT include tremor (i.e., repetitive, regular, rhythmic)	0	1	2	3	4
	6. Lower *(legs, knees, ankles, toes)* e.g., lateral knee movement, foot tapping, heel dropping, foot squirming, inversion and eversion of foot	0	1	2	3	4
TRUNK MOVEMENTS:	7. Neck, shoulders, hips e.g., rocking, twisting, squirming, pelvic gyrations	0	1	2	3	4

GLOBAL JUDGMENTS:	8. Severity of abnormal movements	None, normal Minimal Mild Moderate Severe	0 1 2 3 4
	9. Incapacitation due to abnormal movements	None, normal Minimal Mild Moderate Severe	0 1 2 3 4
	10. Patient's awarness of abnormal movements Rate only patient's report	No awareness Aware, no distress Aware, mild distress Aware, moderate distress Aware, severe distress	0 1 2 3 4

Figure 7.2 *Abnormal involuntary movement scale* (*Source*: Guy W (1976) *ECDEU Assessment Manual for Psychopharmacology*, Rev. National Institute of Mental Health, Rockville, p. 534).

nervous system pathology. In patients who have a history of head trauma or where epilepsy is suspected, a clinical EEG should be done to rule out organic brain disorders (see Table 7.10). When evaluating for epilepsy, several EEGs may be necessary for accurate results because epileptiform activity is not consistently present (Boutros, 1992). The EEG can also play an important role in the diagnosis of dementia, delirium, and other cognitive disorders. Generalized EEG slowing in Alzheimer's dementia is correlated with the degree of cognitive impairment and with decreased regional cerebral blood flow (Hughes and John, 1999). In elderly psychiatric patients, a clinical EEG is of value for distinguishing dementia and pseudodementia associated with depression. This is of

Table 7.9 Common Laboratory Tests for Evaluation of Psychiatric Patients

Serologic
Toxicology screen (blood)
Complete blood count
Blood glucose
Kidney function tests
Liver function tests
Thyroid function tests
Syphilis serology
HIV antibody test
Pregnancy test
Blood cultures
Vitamin B_{12} and folate levels

Urine
Toxicology screen (urine)
Dipstick for protein and glucose
Pregnancy test

Lumbar puncture
Electrocardiogram
Chest radiograph

Table 7.10 Typical Goals of Neuropsychological Testing

Reliably, validly, and as completely as possible, measure the behavioral correlates of brain functions.
Differential diagnosis – identify the characteristic profile associated with a neurobehavioral syndrome.
Establish possible localization, lateralization, and etiology of a brain lesion.
Determine whether neuropsychological deficits are present (i.e., cognitive, perceptual, or motor) regardless of diagnosis.
Describe neuropsychological strengths, weaknesses, and strategy of problem solving.
Assess the patient's feelings about his or her syndrome.
Provide treatment recommendations (i.e., to patient, family, school).

Indications for clinical EEG assessment of psychiatric patients

1. Rule out possible organic brain disorders
2. History of head trauma or suspicion of epilepsy
3. Differentiating pseudodementia secondary to depression and true dementia
4. First presentation of psychosis
5. Pre- and post-electroconvulsive therapy (ECT)
6. Evaluating sleep disorders

importance for treatment selection because EEG abnormality in elderly patients is negatively associated with clinical response to antidepressants (Boutros, 1992).

Patients who experience their first psychotic episode are also candidates for a clinical EEG because brain lesions and seizure disorders, such as temporal lobe epilepsy, can cause psychotic symptoms that are clinically indistinguishable from functional psychoses. EEG recordings before, during, and after ECT for depression also have clinical relevance (Hughes, 1996; Small, 1999). Patients with pretreatment EEG abnormalities may respond less well to ECT (Drake and Shy, 1989), and changes in EEG after ECT generally accompany clinical improvement (Sackeim *et al.*, 1996). Reviews of clinical EEG findings in childhood and adult psychiatric disorders show that 30–60% of referrals have abnormal EEGs (Hughes, 1996; Small, 1999), which underscores the importance of clinical EEG evaluations in psychiatry. One of the limitations of routine clinical EEG is that it is dependent on the trained eye of the reader and is therefore subject to human error and may miss subtle abnormalities in the EEG tracing. Brain potentials evoked by auditory or visual stimuli (e.g., clicks or tones) have been used in both clinical and research contexts in psychiatry. Brain stem evoked potentials (BSEPs) refer to seven positive potentials evoked during the first 12 milliseconds after hearing a click. BSEPs have proven useful for assessment of hearing in infants and uncooperative patients, and in the assessment of brain stem lesions and multiple sclerosis (Celesia and Brigell, 1999). A later event-related P3 or P300 potential, typically recorded during an "oddball" target detection task with either auditory or visual stimuli, refers to a positive potential that peaks 300–500 milliseconds after onset of an infrequent target stimulus. The strongest case for the clinical utility of the P3 potential is in aging and dementia (Polich, 1999). Longer P3 latency distinguishes patients with dementia from those with pseudodementia secondary to depression, and patients with Alzheimer's disease from healthy subjects (Ford *et al.*, 1997; Frodl *et al.*, 2002; Polich and Herbst, 2000). Although P3 provides a useful index of cognitive efficiency, it has little value for the differential diagnosis of psychiatric disorders such as schizophrenia because it lacks specificity.

Brain Imaging

Several methods of brain imaging are available to assist in diagnostic assessment (Table 7.11).

Computed tomography (CT) scans and MRI can be used to assess brain structure and are useful in detecting such abnormalities as mass lesions (central nervous system neoplasms, certain infections, and hemorrhages), calcifications, atrophy, or areas of infarction. Mass lesions should be suspected in situations in which focal or lateralizing abnormalities such as focal weakness, unilateral disturbances in reflexes, and increased pupillary size are found during the neurological examination. Other situations that call for brain imaging include the workup of a patient with dementia to look for brain atrophy or lacunar infarctions; the evaluation of new-onset psychosis, acute onset of aphasia or memory loss, and neglect syndromes; the evaluation of normal-pressure hydrocephalus (a syndrome characterized by a wide-based gait, dementia, and urinary incontinence); and demyelinating conditions.

Whereas CT and MRI provide visualization of brain structure, PET, single photon emission computed tomography (SPECT), and regional cerebral blood flow allow investigators to study brain functioning by assessing which areas of the brain are stimulated during various types of mental activity.

Table 7.11 Indications for Brain Imaging
History of head trauma
Focal neurological findings on physical examination
New-onset psychosis
New-onset psychiatric symptoms after age 40 (including affective disorder and personality change)
Rapid onset of psychiatric symptoms
History of neurological symptoms (including seizures)
Evidence of cognitive impairment
Abnormal electroencephalogram
Abnormal lumbar puncture

Special Assessment Techniques

In certain situations, special assessment techniques may be indicated in the psychiatric evaluation of patients who are unable or unwilling to cooperate. These situations include the assessment of patients who are mute, have amnesia, or intentionally provide false information. In general, special techniques are employed only after all conventional ways to obtain the necessary information have been exhausted, including the use of other informants where available and appropriate.

Hypnosis can aid in the recovery of repressed memories. For example, a patient who presents with a conversion symptom may be able to recall the forgotten traumatic events that precipitated it. The usefulness of hypnosis is limited by the patient's susceptibility to the procedure and by concern that the interviewer's suggestions can produce false memories.

Another approach available for similar purposes is to use a sedative during the interview to produce disinhibition and allow the patient to speak more freely or access otherwise unavailable memories. Intravenous amobarbital sodium is the best known of the medications used for this purpose. Caution must be exercised to avoid oversedation, to monitor for side effects of the medication, and to ensure that the interviewer does not inappropriately influence the patient's answers.

Treatment Planning

The psychiatric evaluation is the basis for developing the case formulation, initial treatment plan, initial disposition, and comprehensive treatment plan.

Case Formulation

The case formulation is the summary statement of the immediate problem, the context in which the problem has arisen, the tentative diagnosis, and the assessment of risk. The latter two areas are described next in more detail.

Assessment of Risk

The assessment of risk is the most crucial component of the formulation because the safety of the patient, the clinician, and others is the foremost concern in any psychiatric evaluation. Four areas are important: suicide risk, assault risk, life-threatening medical conditions, and external threat.

Suicide Risk

The risk of suicide is the most common life-threatening situation mental health professionals encounter. Its assessment is based on both an understanding of its epidemiology, which alerts the clinician to potential danger, and the individualized assessment of the patient. Suicide is the eighth leading cause of death in the USA. In the past century, the rate of suicide has averaged 12.5 per 100,000 people. Studies of adults and adolescents who commit suicide reveal that more than 90% of them suffered from at least one psychiatric disorder and as many as 80% of them consulted a physician in the months preceding the event. An astute risk assessment therefore provides an opportunity for prevention.

For those who complete suicide, the most common diagnoses are affective disorder (45–70%) and alcoholism (25%). In certain psychiatric disorders, there is a significant lifetime risk for suicide, as listed in Table 7.12. Panic disorder is associated with an elevated rate of suicidal ideation and suicide attempts, but estimates of rates of completed suicide are not well established.

Table 7.12 Estimated Lifetime Rates of Completed Suicide by Diagnosis
Major affective disorders: 10–15%
Alcoholism: 10–15% (comorbid depression usually present)
Schizophrenia: 10% (often during a post-psychotic depressive state)
Borderline and antisocial personality disorders: 5–10%

Suicide rates increase with age, although rates among young adults have been steadily rising. Women attempt suicide more often than men, but men are three to four times more likely than women to complete suicide. Whites have higher rates of suicide than other groups.

A patient may fit the diagnostic and demographic profile for suicide risk, but even more essential is the individualized assessment developed by integrating information from all parts of the psychiatric evaluation. This includes material from the present illness (e.g., symptoms of depression, paranoid ideation about being harmed), past psychiatric history (e.g., prior attempts at suicide or other violent behavior), personal history (e.g., recent loss), family history (e.g., suicide or violence in close relatives), medical history (e.g., presence of a terminal illness), and the MSE (e.g., helplessness, suicidal ideation).

The most consistent predictor of future suicidal behavior is a prior history of such behavior, which is especially worrisome when previous suicide attempts have involved serious intent or lethal means. Among the factors cited as having an association with risk of suicide are current use of drugs and alcohol; recent loss, such as of a spouse or job; social isolation; conduct disorders and antisocial behavior, especially in young men; the presence of depression, especially when it is accompanied by hopelessness, helplessness, delusions, or agitation; certain psychotic symptoms, such as command hallucinations and frightening paranoid delusions; fantasies of reunion by death; and severe medical illness, especially when it is associated with loss of functioning, intractable pain, or central nervous system dysfunction. Table 7.13 lists risk factors for suicide. Depression

Table 7.13 Risk Factors for Suicide

Category	Risk Factors for Suicide
Demographic	White Male Older age Divorced, never married, or widowed Unemployed
Historical	Previous suicide attempts, especially with serious intent, lethal means, or disappointment about survival Family history of suicide Victim of physical or sexual abuse
Psychiatric	Diagnosis: affective disorder, alcoholism, panic disorder, psychotic disorders, conduct disorder, severe personality disorder (especially antisocial and borderline) Symptoms: suicidal or homicidal ideation; depression, especially with hopelessness, helplessness, anhedonia, delusions, agitation; mixed mania and depression; psychotic symptoms, including command hallucinations and persecutory delusions Current use of alcohol or illicit drugs Recent psychiatric hospitalization
Environmental	Recent loss such as that of a spouse or job Social isolation Access to guns or other lethal weapons Social acceptance of suicide
Medical	Severe medical illness, especially with loss of functioning or intractable pain Delirium or confusion caused by central nervous system dysfunction
Behavioral	Antisocial acts Poor impulse control, risk taking, and aggressiveness Preparing for death (e.g., making a will, giving away possessions, stockpiling lethal medication) Well-developed, detailed suicide plan Statements of intent to inflict harm on self or others

is a strong predictor of suicidal ideation. Among those with suicidal ideation, anxiety disorders predict suicide attempts.

It is essential to be clear about whether the patient has passive thoughts about suicide or actual intent. Is there a plan? If so, how detailed is it, how lethal, and what are the chances of rescue? The possession of firearms is particularly worrisome, because nearly two-thirds of documented suicides among men and more than a third among women have involved firearms.

Factors that may protect against suicide include convictions in opposition to suicide; strong attachments to others, including spouse and children; and evidence of good impulse control.

Risk of Assault

Unlike those who commit suicide, most people who commit violent acts have not been diagnosed with a mental illness, and data clarifying the relationship between mental illness and violence are limited. The most common psychiatric diagnoses associated with violence are substance-related disorders. Conduct disorder and antisocial personality disorder, by definition, involve aggressive, violent, and/or unlawful behavior.

In the absence of comorbid substance-related disorders, most people with such major mental illnesses as affective disorders and schizophrenia are not violent. But data from the National Institute of Mental Health Epidemiological Catchment Area Study suggest that these diagnoses are associated with a higher rate of violence than that found among individuals who have no diagnosable mental illness. The MacArthur Violence Risk Assessment Study found this was only true for psychiatric patients with substance abuse (Steadman *et al.*, 1998).

Table 7.14 lists risk factors for violence. As with suicide, the best predictor of future assault is a history of past assault. Information from the psychiatric evaluation that helps in this assessment includes the present illness (e.g., preoccupation with vengeance, especially when accompanied by a plan of action), psychiatric history (e.g., childhood conduct disorder), family history (e.g., exposure as a child to violent parental behavior), personal history (e.g., arrest record), and the MSE (e.g., homicidal ideation, severe agitation). Other predictors of violence include possession of weapons and current illegal activities. There is considerable overlap between risk factors for suicide and those for violence.

External Threat

Some patients who present for psychiatric evaluation are at risk of life-threatening external situations. Such patients include battered women, abused children, and victims of catastrophes who lack proper food or shelter. Information about these conditions is usually obtained from the present illness, the personal history, the medical history, and physical examination.

Table 7.14 Risk Factors for Violence

Category	Risk Factors
Demographic	Young Male Limited education Unemployed
Historical	Previous history of violence to self or others, especially with high degree of lethality History of animal torture Past antisocial or criminal behavior Violence within family of origin Victim of physical or sexual abuse
Psychiatric	Diagnosis: substance-related disorders, antisocial personality disorder; conduct disorder; intermittent explosive disorder; pathological alcohol intoxication; psychoses (e.g., paranoid, toxic) Symptoms: physical agitation; intent to kill or take revenge; identification of specific victim(s); psychotic symptoms, especially command hallucinations to commit violence and persecutory delusions Current use of alcohol or other drugs
Environmental	Access to guns or other lethal weapons Living under circumstances of violence Membership in violent group
Medical	Delirium or confusion caused by central nervous system dysfunction Disinhibition caused by traumatic brain injuries and other central nervous system dysfunctions Toxic states related to metabolic disorders (e.g., hyperthyroidism)
Behavioral	Antisocial acts Agitation, anger Poor impulse control; risk taking or reckless behavior Statements of intent to inflict harm

Differential Diagnosis

The differential diagnosis is best approached by organizing the information obtained in the psychiatric evaluation into five domains of mental functioning according to the disturbances revealed by the evaluation (see Table 7.15). After organizing the information into these five domains, the psychiatrist looks for the psychopathological syndromes and potential diagnoses that best account for the disturbances described.

Table 7.15 Categorizing Features of Mental Disturbance

Area of Mental Functioning	Examples of Relevant Evidence of Disturbance
Consciousness, orientation, and memory	Abnormalities on interview or MSE, especially impairments in awareness; alertness; orientation to person, place, time; immediate, short-term, or long-term memory; attention; calculations; fund of knowledge; abstractions Past history of foregoing Positive substance use history Risk factors for HIV; positive HIV antibody result Focal neurological findings on physical examination Laboratory and brain imaging abnormalities Impairments on neuropsychological testing
Speech, thinking, perception, and self-experience	Abnormalities on interview or MSE, especially disturbances of speech, thinking, reality testing, and presence of hallucinations, delusions Past history of foregoing
Emotions	Abnormalities on interview or MSE, especially labile, depressed, expansive, elevated, irritable mood, and inappropriate affect, anger, or anxiety Past history of foregoing Positive scores for mood disturbance on structured interviews
Physical signs and symptoms; physiological disturbances	Physical or neurological findings indicative of medical or mental disorder Laboratory abnormalities Past medical illnesses Positive substance use history
Behavior and adaptive functioning	Personality dysfunction Impaired social or occupational functioning Impaired activities of daily living Impulsive, compulsive, or avoidant behaviors History of behavioral or functional disturbances Personal history (highest levels of achievement)

A complete diagnostic evaluation includes assessments on each of the five axes of DSM-IV-TR (Table 7.16).

Disturbances of consciousness, orientation, and memory are most typically associated with delirium related to a general medical condition or a substance use disorder. Memory impairment and other cognitive disturbances are the hallmarks of dementia. Results of the history, physical examination, laboratory testing, and brain imaging often help in defining the specific etiology. It is important to elicit risk factors for HIV infection and, when they are present, to encourage voluntary HIV antibody testing.

Table 7.16 DSM-IV-TR Multiaxial System

Axis I	Clinical disorders
	Other conditions that may be a focus of clinical attention
Axis II	Personality disorders
	Mental retardation
Axis III	General medical conditions
Axis IV	Psychosocial and environmental problems
Axis V	Global assessment of functioning

Neuropsychological testing is particularly useful in the diagnosis of subcortical dementia, such as that caused by Huntington's disease and HIV infection. Dissociative disorders and severe psychotic states may also present with disturbances in this domain without evidence of any medical etiology. Cognitive impairment caused by mental retardation is established by intelligence testing.

Disturbances of speech, thinking, perception, and self-experience are common in psychotic states that can be seen in patients with such diagnoses as schizophrenia and mania, as well as in central nervous system dysfunction caused by substance use or a medical condition. Disturbances in self-experience are also common in dissociative disorders and certain anxiety, somatoform, and eating disorders. Cluster A personality disorders may be associated with milder forms of disturbances in this domain (American Psychiatric Association, 2000).

Disturbances of emotion are most typical of affective and anxiety disorders. These disturbances may also be caused by substance use disorders and general medical conditions. Mood and affect disturbances accompany many personality disorders and may be especially pronounced in borderline personality disorder.

Physical signs and symptoms and any associated abnormalities revealed by diagnostic medical tests and past medical history are used to establish the presence of general medical conditions, which are coded on Axis III. When a medical disorder is causally related to a psychiatric disorder, a statement of this relationship should appear on Axis I. Physical signs and symptoms may also suggest diagnoses of mood or anxiety disorders or states of substance intoxication or withdrawal. Physical symptoms for which no medical etiology can be demonstrated after thorough assessment suggest somatoform or factitious disorders or malingering, although the possibility of an as-yet-undiagnosed medical condition should still be kept in mind.

Information about behavior and adaptive functioning is useful for diagnosing personality disorders, documenting psychosocial and environmental problems on Axis IV, and assessing global functioning on Axis V. This information is also useful for diagnosing most psychiatric disorders, which typically include criteria related to abnormal behaviors and functional impairment.

When all information has been gathered and organized, it may be possible to reach definitive diagnoses, but sometimes this must await further evaluation and the development of the comprehensive treatment plan.

Initial Treatment Plan

The initial treatment plan follows the case formulation, which has already established the nature of the current problem and a tentative diagnosis. The plan distinguishes between what must be accomplished now and what is postponed for the future. Treatment planning works best when it follows the biopsychosocial model.

Biological Intervention

This includes an immediate response to any life-threatening medical conditions and a plan for the treatment of other less acute physical disorders, including those that may contribute to an altered mental status. Prescription of psychotropic medications in accordance with the tentative diagnosis is the most common biological intervention.

Psychosocial Intervention

This includes immediate plans to prevent violent or suicidal behavior and address adverse external circumstances. An overall strategy must be developed that is both realistic and responsive to the patient's situation. Developing this strategy requires an awareness of the social support systems available to the patient; the financial resources of the patient; the availability of services in the area; the need to contact other agencies, such as child welfare or the police; and the need to ensure child care for dependent children.

Initial Disposition

The primary task of the initial disposition is to select the most appropriate level of care after completion of the psychiatric evaluation. Disposition is primarily focused on immediate goals. After referral, the patient and the treatment team develop longer-term goals. The first decision in any disposition plan is whether hospitalization is required to ensure safety. There are times when a patient presents with such severe risk of harm to self or others that hospitalization seems essential. In other cases, the patient could be managed outside the hospital, depending on the availability of other supports. This might include a family who can stay with the patient or a crisis team in the community able to treat the patient at home. The more comprehensive the system of services, the easier it is to avoid hospitalization. Because hospitalization is associated with extreme disruption of usual life activities and in and of itself can have many adverse consequences, plans to avoid hospitalization are usually appropriate as long as they do not compromise safety.

The most common referral after psychiatric evaluation is to psychotherapy and/or medication management. In office-based settings, the psychiatrist decides whether he or she has the time and expertise to treat the patient and makes referrals to other practitioners as appropriate. Hospital staff usually have a broad overview of community resources and refer accordingly. There are high rates of dropout when patients are sent from one setting to another. These can be reduced by providing introductions to the treatment setting and/or conducting follow-up to ensure that the referral has been successful.

Table 7.17 Areas Covered by Comprehensive Treatment Plan

Mental health
Diagnoses on five axes
Psychiatric management, including medications
Physical health
Medical diagnoses
Medical management, including medications
Personal strengths and assets
Rehabilitation needs
Educational
Occupational
Social
Activities of daily living skills
Use of leisure time
Living arrangements
Social supports and family involvement
Finances
Personal finances
Insurance coverage
Eligibility for social service benefits
Legal or forensic issues
Central goals and objectives
Listing of treatment team members
Evidence of participation by patient and, as appropriate, family members and others
Criteria for discharge from treatment

The comprehensive treatment plan usually includes more definitive diagnoses and a well-formulated management plan with central goals and objectives. For severely ill or hospitalized patients, every area is usually covered (Table 7.17). It is best for the patient and, as appropriate, the family to have input into the plan. The comprehensive treatment plan guides and coordinates the direction of all treatment for an extended time, usually months, and is periodically reviewed and updated. For more focal psychiatric problems (e.g., phobias, sexual dysfunctions) and more limited interventions (e.g., brief interpersonal, cognitive, and behavioral therapies in office-based practices), the comprehensive treatment plan may focus on only several of the possible areas.

Conclusion

The psychiatric evaluation is a method of collecting present and past psychological, biological, social, and environmental data for the purpose of establishing a comprehensive picture of the patient's strengths and problems, including the psychiatric diagnoses, and developing treatment plans. It is the essential beginning of every course of psychiatric treatment and, when carried out successfully, integrates a multimodal approach to understanding mental illness and providing clinical care.

References

American Psychiatric Association (2000) *Diagnostic and Statistical Manual of Mental Disorders*, 4th edn, Text Rev.APA, Washington, DC.

Boutros NN (1992) A review of indications for routine EEG in clinical psychiatry. *Hospital & Community Psychiatry* 43, 716–719.

Celesia GG and Brigell MG (1999) Auditory evoked potentials, in *Electroencephalography: Basic Principles, Clinical Applications, and Related Fields*, 4th edn (eds Niedermeyer E and Lopes Da Silva F). Lippincott, Williams & Wilkins, Baltimore, pp. 994–1013.

Council on Scientific Affairs (1987) Scientific issues in drug testing. *Journal of American Medical Association* 257, 3110–3114.

Drake ME and Shy KE (1989) Predictive value of electroencephalography for electroconvulsive therapy. *Clinical Electroencephalography* 20, 55–57.

Ford JM, Roth WT, Isaacks BG *et al.* (1997) Automatic and effortful processing in aging and dementia: Event-related brain potentials. *Neurobiology of Aging* 18, 169–180.

Frodl T, Hampel H, Juckel G *et al.* (2002) Value of event related P300 subcomponents in the clinical diagnosis of mild cognitive impairment and Alzheimer's Disease. *Psychophysiology* 39, 175–181.

Gold MS and Dackis CA (1986) Role of the laboratory in the evaluation of suspected drug abuse. *The Journal of Clinical Psychiatry* 47(Suppl.), 17–23.

Hughes JR (1996) A review of the usefulness of the standard EEG in psychiatry. *Clinical Electroencephalography* 27, 35–39.

Hughes JR and John ER (1999) Conventional and quantitative electroencephalography in psychiatry. *The Journal of Neuropsychiatry and Clinical Neurosciences* 11, 190–207.

Polich J (1999) P300 in clinical applications, in *Electroencephalography: Basic Principles, Clinical Applications and Related Fields*, 4th edn (eds Niedermeyer E and Lopes Da Silva F). Lippincott, Williams & Wilkins, Baltimore, pp. 1073–1091.

Polich J and Herbst KL (2000) P300 as a clinical assay: Rationale, evaluation, and findings. *International Journal of Psychophysiology* 38, 3–19.

Sackeim HA, Luber B, Katzman GP *et al.* (1996) The effects of electroconvulsive therapy on quantitative electroencephalograms. *Archives of General Psychiatry* 53, 814–824.

Small JG (1999) Psychiatric disorders and EEG, in *Electroencephalography: Basic Principles, Clinical Applications, and Related Fields*, 4th edn (eds Niedermeyer E and Lopes Da Silva F). Lippincott, Williams & Wilkins, Baltimore, pp. 603–620.

Steadman HJ, Gounis K, Dennis D *et al.* (1998) Violence by people discharged from acute psychiatric inpatient facilities and by others in the same neighborhoods. *Archives of General Psychiatry* 55, 393–401.

CHAPTER

8 Professional Ethics and Boundaries

Introduction

In the last several decades, advances in psychiatry have made it possible to treat mental disorders that were previously unamenable to successful intervention. There has been a dark side to this progress, however, because futuristic anticipation of subduing disease and forcing nature to surrender her secrets has led many practitioners to outrun their headlights. Like technical sorcerers of science fiction confusing promise with reality, we are in danger of being lulled into an intellectual arrogance that can cause us to forget what it means to be professionals. One manifestation of this process has been the defensive reliance by clinicians on reductionistic explanations for complex and multidetermined disorders, combined with a neglect of the important role of trust and empathy as a curative factor in treating mental disorders.

A bewildering potpourri of treatment options and methods for financing health care presents psychiatrists with other sources of confusion. Patients' health and safety often depend upon our ability to make rapid clinical decisions regarding diagnosis and to utilize an optimal psychotherapeutic or psychopharmacologic approach. The psychiatrist's dilemma is similarly compounded by conflicts between the cost-determined restrictions of managed care and the sacred promise to advocate primarily for patients' welfare.

Building a cooperative and trusting relationship with patients has always been an essential factor enabling clinicians to foster the healing process. In ancient times, when there were few specific remedies available, physicians relied on a highly integrative view of the sick person. In most instances, modern technology augments but cannot substitute for a trusting doctor–patient relationship. Patients seeking medical care must suspend ordinary social distance and critical judgment if they are to allow physicians to enter their physical and psychological space. As we review in this chapter, the ability to sustain a professional attitude and to practice within a set of coherent boundaries forms the foundation of proper psychiatric treatment, regardless of theoretic orientation or treatment modality. An understanding of psychiatric ethics plays a vital role in the psychiatrist's ability to keep proper boundaries because these values provide a stable beacon in the cognitively perplexing fog that so often pervades the treatment situation.

The Psychiatric Interview: Evaluation and Diagnosis, First Edition. Allan Tasman, Jerald Kay and Robert J. Ursano.

This chapter is based on Chapter 5 (Richard S. Epstein, Ahmed Okasha) of *Psychiatry*, 3rd Edition.

Ethical Behavior and Its Relationship to the Professional Attitude

In modern times, a professional is expected to be a learned person who has acquired special knowledge of a subject that is of vital importance for the welfare of the community. Having expertise is not enough, however. A professional is also obliged to adhere to certain societal responsibilities that are founded upon a code of ethical behavior and an attitude of service to those in need. A professional commitment to ethical behavior and service must take precedence over monetary compensation. All physicians, including psychiatrists, are bound by such a covenant – a sacred vow to place patient well-being before other considerations. In Western medical tradition, this obligation primarily derives from the teachings of Hippocrates in the 5th century BC. The Hippocratic Oath is often recited at the graduation exercises of American medical schools. It includes three of the six core principles of modern medical ethics: *beneficence*, *nonmalfeasance*, and *confidentiality*:

> I will follow that system of regimen which according to my ability and judgment, I consider for the benefit of my patients, and abstain from whatever is deleterious and mischievous.... With purity and holiness I will pass my life and practice my Art.... Into whatever houses I enter, I will go into them for the benefit of the sick, and will abstain from every voluntary act of mischief and corruption; and, further, from the seduction of females or males, of freemen and slaves. Whatever, in connection with my professional practice or not, in connection with it, I see or hear, in the life of men, which ought not to be spoken of abroad, I will not divulge, as reckoning that all such should be kept secret. (Hippocrates, 1929)

The other three general principles of medical ethics include autonomy, justice, and veracity (see Table 8.1 for a description and summary of all six ethical principles; Epstein, 1994, p. 20). The American Psychiatric Association (APA) (1973) adopted the American Medical Association's (AMA) *Principles of Medical Ethics*, publishing it along with special annotations applicable for psychiatric practice. The APA has produced six revisions

Table 8.1 Six Basic Principles of Medical Ethics

Principle	Description
Beneficence	Applying one's abilities solely for the patient's well-being
Nonmalfeasance	Avoiding harm to a patient
Autonomy	Respect for a patient's independence
Justice	Avoiding prejudicial bias based on idiosyncrasies of the patient's background, behavior, or station in life
Confidentiality	Respect for the patient's privacy
Veracity	Truthfulness with oneself and one's patients

Source: Epstein (1994). Reprinted with permission from *Keeping Boundaries: Maintaining Safety and Integrity in the Psychotherapeutic Process*, Text Revision. Copyright 1994, American Psychiatric Association, Washington, DC.

of these annotations. The seven sections of the AMA principles are summarized in Table 8.2. Table 8.3 summarizes some of the salient ethical annotations for psychiatrists (American Psychiatric Association, 1993).

Table 8.2 Summary of the Principles of Ethics of the American Medical Association

Section	Statement of Principle
Preamble	The medical profession's ethical standards are designed primarily for the well-being of patients. As professionals, physicians are required to acknowledge a responsibility to patients, to society, to self, and to their colleagues.
Section I	Dedication to competent, compassionate care. Respect for human dignity.
Section II	Obligation to deal honestly with patients and colleagues and to expose physicians who are incompetent or fraudulent.
Section III	Respect for the law. Obligation to seek changes in laws harmful to patient's care.
Section IV	Respect for the rights of patients and colleagues. Within legal constraints, preservation of confidentiality.
Section V	Commitment to continued education, sharing of relevant knowledge, and obtaining necessary consultation.
Section VI	Except in emergency, freedom to decide whom to treat, with whom to associate, and the setting in which one serves.
Section VII	Acknowledge the responsibility to contribute to improving the community.

Source: American Psychiatric Association (1993) *Principles of Medical Ethics with Annotations Especially Applicable to Psychiatry*. Copyright, American Psychiatric Association, Washington DC.

Table 8.3 Summary of Selected Ethical Principles for Psychiatrists

Principle	Annotations
Competent care	The psychiatrist must scrutinize the effect of his or her conduct on the boundaries of the treatment relationship.
Honest dealing	Sex with a current or former patient is unethical. Information given by patients should not be exploited. Contractual arrangements should be explicit. Fee splitting is unethical.
Confidentiality, respecting colleagues	Restraint in release of information to third parties. Adequate disguise of case presentations. Disclosure of lack of confidentiality in nontreatment situations. Sex with students or supervisees may be unethical.

Source: American Psychiatric Association (1993) *Principles of Medical Ethics with Annotations Especially Applicable to Psychiatry*. Copyright, American Psychiatric Association, Washington, DC.

The World Psychiatric Association developed and approved ethical guidelines, starting with the Declaration of Hawaii in 1977, galvanized by concerns about the abuse of psychiatry. A long process of investigation within the domain of professional ethics provided the foundation for the Declaration of Madrid that was endorsed by the General Assembly of the WPA in 1996. In its final form, the Declaration of Madrid included seven general guidelines that focused on the aims of psychiatry. They are summarized as follows:

1. Psychiatry's concern should be to provide the best treatment and rehabilitation for persons with mental disorders, consistent with scientific knowledge, ethical principles, and with the least possible restriction on the freedom of the patient.
2. Psychiatrists have a duty to keep abreast of scientific developments. Psychiatrists trained in research should seek to advance the frontiers of knowledge.
3. The psychiatrist–patient relationship must be based on mutual trust and respect, and should allow the patient to make free and informed decisions. The psychiatrist has a duty to accept the patient as a partner in the therapy and to empower the patient with necessary information for rational treatment decisions.
4. Psychiatrists should consult with families of incapacitated patients to safeguard the human dignity and the legal rights of the patient. Treatment should not be given against the patient's will, unless withholding treatment would endanger the life of the patient or others. Treatment must always be in the best interest of the patient.
5. Psychiatrists performing assessments, especially when retained by a third party, have a duty to inform the person being examined about the purpose of the intervention, the use of the findings, and the possible repercussions of the assessment.
6. Unless there is a threat of serious harm to the patient or other persons, psychiatrists should keep all patient information in confidence, and use such information only for the purpose of helping the patient. Psychiatrists are prohibited from making use of such information for personal, financial, or academic benefits.
7. It is unethical to conduct research that is not in accordance with the canons of science. Research activities should be approved by an appropriate and ethically constituted oversight committee. Because of the vulnerability of psychiatric patients, extra caution and strict ethical standards should be employed to safeguard patients' autonomy, patients' mental and physical integrity, and the selection of population groups.

An appendix to the Declaration of Madrid includes additional guidelines on specific ethical issues in psychiatry, including the following (World Psychiatric Association Ethical Statements, 2000).

WPA Guidelines on Euthanasia

The physician's role, first and foremost, is to promote health, reduce suffering, and protect life. The psychiatrist, whose patients may include those who are severely incapacitated or incompetent to reach an informal decision, should be particularly careful about actions that could lead to the death of individuals who cannot protect themselves because of disability, and should be vigilant to the possibility that a patient's views could be distorted by mental illness such as depression. In such situations, the psychiatrist's role is to treat the illness.

WPA Guidelines on Torture

A psychiatrist should not take part in any process of mental or physical torture even when authorities attempt to force their involvement in such acts. Furthermore, a psychiatrist should not participate under any circumstances in legally authorized executions, nor participate in assessments of competency to be executed.

WPA Guidelines on Sex Selection

It is unethical for a psychiatrist to participate in decisions to terminate pregnancy for the purpose of sex selection.

WPA Guidelines on Organ Transplantation

Psychiatrists should seek to protect their patients and help them exercise self-determination to the fullest extent possible. The role of the psychiatrist is to clarify the issues surrounding organ donations and to deal with the religious, cultural, social, and family factors to ensure that informed and proper decisions be made by all concerned.

WPA Guidelines on Genetic Research and Counseling in Psychiatric Patients

Psychiatrists participating in genetic research should be mindful that the ramifications of genetic information are not limited to the individual subject or patient but can lead to far-reaching repercussions and consequences that can have a negative and disruptive effect on the larger family or community. Psychiatrists are ethically obligated to observe proper practice, avoid the risks associated with premature disclosure, misinterpretations, or misuse of genetic information, and should never advise a pregnant woman with mental disorders to get an abortion based on the medical or genetic basis of her mental illness. They should not refer patients to genetic testing unless there are satisfactory levels of quality assurance and adequate genetic counseling available to the patient.

Further guidelines on the relationship between psychiatrists and the media, ethnic discrimination, ethnic cleansing, and genetic research and counseling were endorsed by the WPA General Assembly in 1999.

WPA Guidelines on Ethnic Discrimination and Ethnic Cleansing

The Madrid Declaration defines ethnic discrimination as basically racist, as it fails to accept diversity and humanity's common heritage. In its most malignant form, ethnic cleansing is a crime against humanity. In this regard, psychiatrists should not discriminate nor help to discriminate against patients on ethnic grounds, nor be involved in any activity that promotes ethnic cleansing.

WPA Guidelines on Psychiatrists Addressing the Media

It is important that psychiatrists use the media in an affirmative way for a variety of goals that promote good mental health care, such as advocating for the destigmatization of mental disorder and mental patients. In all their interactions with the media, psychiatrists are obliged to advocate for the mentally ill and to maintain the dignity of the profession. Psychiatrists should be mindful of the effect of their statements on the public perception of the profession and patients, and abstain from making statements or undertaking public activities that may be demeaning to either. Patients' confidentiality should be maintained, and the sensationalization of mental illness should be avoided. Regarding the disclosure of research findings, psychiatrists should be cautious to report only results that are generally accepted by experts, and to convey the presentation of such results in a way that serves patients' welfare and dignity.

The Coherent Treatment Frame and the Role of Therapeutic Boundaries in Effective Psychiatric Treatment

The "frame" of a social interaction was defined by Goffman (1974) as consisting of the spoken and unspoken expectations defining meaning and involvement in a given situation. For example, patients seek out psychiatrists based on a tacit assumption that the doctor is a reliable and experienced clinician who has the ability to assist them in finding relief for distress. However, many patients tend to frame their treatment in pathological ways. For example, some will attempt to pressure the psychiatrist into the role of a magical wizard who will confer unconditional love and pleasure. Whatever method the patient employs to frame the relationship, any abrupt disappointment or rupture of these unspoken expectations often results in intense and disruptive feelings of mortification and betrayal. A sudden breach of a social frame can lead to the dissolution of one's sense of meaning and connection, and is often accompanied by intense feelings of shame.

The psychiatrist's task is to provide a coherent therapeutic frame within which to contain the patient's illness. The psychiatrist's frame makes it secure to proceed with the specific therapeutic modality, just as the surgical suite provides a safe environment for operative techniques. The treatment frame enables the patient to maintain a feeling of trust and connectedness while learning to deal with the unrealistic nature of his or her expectations. The frame comprises various boundary factors that include acting in a reliable way, showing respect for the patient's autonomy by explaining the potential risks and benefits of the treatment method, maintaining confidentiality, avoiding exploitation of the patient's sexual feelings, and resisting the patient's manipulative efforts by explaining the maladaptive nature of such behavior.

Boundary Violations

Psychiatric treatment cannot be conducted without doctor and patient entering into each other's space, just as it is impossible to perform a bloodless laparotomy. Many patients are unable to articulate their sense of injury because the psychiatrist's aberrant behavior may appear so similar to exploitation they have experienced in previous pathological relationships. For example, patients who were sexually abused in childhood are more likely to acquiesce to an amorous advance by a psychiatrist and to avoid complaining about feeling used, because they fear the threat of the psychiatrist's rejection and retaliation. Certain nonsexual boundary crossings such as conflicts of interest might seem harmless on the surface but can interfere with patients' ability to feel safe in their psychiatrist's care and will diminish their chances for optimal recovery. In this context, a boundary violation can be defined as any infringement that interferes with the primary goal of providing care or causes harm to the patient, the therapist, or the therapy itself.

The public has become increasingly interested in the subject of psychiatric boundary violations in the past 25 years, particularly those involving sexual exploitation. State licensing boards, professional ethics committees, and civil juries are much more likely to mete out strong sanctions against violators than ever before. These attitudinal changes have taken place in spite of the fact that popular movies continue to romanticize the idea of psychiatrist–patient sexuality, and almost always seem oblivious to the horrendous feelings of shame, betrayal, and devastation that patients experience when these things happen to them in real life.

The public's intolerance of sexual involvement between psychiatrists and patients has resulted in part from the increasing empowerment of the victims of incest, rape, and spousal abuse, and a better understanding of the psychological sequelae that follow mental trauma such as posttraumatic stress disorder (PTSD). In addition, psychiatric patients have become more willing to expose unethical or exploitative behavior on the part of clinicians, particularly when it involves sexual activity. This trend has been augmented by the fact that courts and professional licensing bodies are now more inclined to render sanctions for injuries that are solely psychological in nature.

When clinicians engage in nonsexual infringements of the treatment relationship, it may be a prelude to subsequent sexual behavior. Sexual involvement with patients often starts with excessive personal disclosure, accepting and giving gifts, requesting favors, and meeting patients outside of the office setting. Regardless of the specific type of infringement involved, there are common elements to all boundary violations, including efforts on the part of the clinician to reverse roles with the patient, to intimidate the patient to maintain secrecy, to place the patient in a double bind, and to indulge professional privilege. Indulgence of privilege is often accompanied by a sense of entitlement on the clinician's part, such that he or she regards the patient as a wholly owned subsidiary. Circumstances impairing the clinician's ability to cope with patients and their problems may include deficient knowledge, general stress, mental disorder, or a treatment-induced regression. These factors may lead the clinician to employ maladaptive intrapsychic or behavioral coping mechanisms that manifest in the form of therapeutic boundary violations. Other general factors are common to all boundary violations.

An exploitive therapist blurs the logical boundaries between the two subcategories and fails to inform the patient that sexual behavior with him is likely to be harmful to her. Blurring of logical categories is an essential aspect of double-binding messages. Patients who are subjected to such reasoning are often in a dependent and cognitively regressed state and are unable to understand the logical absurdity of the double bind. They fear that if they refuse to comply with the therapist's suggestions, they will be rejected for failing to cooperate with the therapist.

It is important to place the burgeoning literature on boundary violations in its social context. The public has recently been more often hearing reports of psychiatrists and other mental health professionals who have been disciplined or sued for behavior such as sexual involvement with patients and spouses of patients, using information learned in patients' psychotherapy sessions to gain inside data on financial investments, and accepting large bequests from patients.

Components of the Coherent Psychiatric Frame

The purpose of the therapeutic frame is to protect the patient's safety and to promote recovery. It is the therapist's responsibility to structure the frame through word and deed. A healthy and secure therapeutic environment is predicated on reducing variability and uncertainty in the treatment setting as much as possible. Table 8.4 summarizes the major boundary factors comprising the coherent treatment frame. Careful attention to these boundary issues can assist treating psychiatrists to communicate defining messages that strengthen the differentiation of role and identity between patient and practitioner.

Just as the diversity of opinion regarding optimal methods of treatment for specific psychiatric disorders makes it very difficult to devise a set of specific guidelines that are appropriate for psychiatrists adhering to a wide spectrum of theoretical orientations, there is diversity in defining a comprehensive ethical system, whether it is based on a set of specific rules (deontological ethics), on a list of values and goals (teleological ethics), or from consideration of the emotional and practical consequences of a given course of action (consequentialist ethics). A parallel dilemma exists when it comes to defining psychiatric boundaries. For this reason, guidelines for psychiatrists should enhance patient safety, foster adherence to established clinical principles, and help to avoid specific consequences that are detrimental to either patient or practitioner. Such an approach is consistent with an intensifying interest in reducing preventable medical error.

Table 8.4 Major Boundary Issues Contributing to the Formation of a Coherent Treatment Frame

Boundary Issue	Function and Purpose	Implicit Message to Patient
Stability	Consistency as to time, place, location, parties involved, and treatment method	"The doctor is reliable. This treatment can contain my irrationality".
Avoiding dual relationships	Utmost fidelity to the primary purpose of helping the patient	"The doctor focuses his or her attention on my problem, and is not sidetracked".
Neutrality and promoting patient autonomy	Avoiding abuse of power and promoting the patient's independence	"The doctor values my ideas and encourages me to exercise choices".
Noncollusive compensation	Scrupulous and forthright terms of remuneration for the clinician	"Aside from the payment, I don't have to gratify the doctor".
Confidentiality	To protect the patient's privilege of keeping his or her communications secret	"My thoughts and feelings belong to me, not to the doctor".
Anonymity	Avoids seductiveness and role reversal	"This is a place to bring my issues, not a forum for the doctor's personal problems".
Abstinence	Encourages verbalization rather than action in dealing with feelings and conflicts	"There is a big difference between wishes and reality".
Preserving the clinician's safety and self-respect	Discourages the patient's destructive behavior, sets a good role model for establishing healthy self-esteem	"It is possible to have a close relationship without someone getting hurt".

Stability

Patients with psychiatric illnesses will find it very difficult to entrust their lives to a psychiatrist whom they perceive to be unreliable. Indicated measures regarding stability include formulating an agreement with the patient for a treatment regimen that will take place according to a specific method and schedule, encouraging truthful disclosure and cooperation, establishing a commitment to beginning and ending sessions on time, discouraging interruptions during treatment sessions, offering advance notice as to when the psychiatrist will be absent, providing for coverage by another practitioner when the psychiatrist is off duty, maintaining coherent therapeutic demeanor, and maintaining relative consistency as to who participates in the treatment situation.

It is generally unwise for a psychiatrist to disparage a patient's complaints about issues like the doctor's tardiness in starting sessions or to become defensive when explaining the meaning of the patient's distress about such complaints. Many psychiatrists experience patients' demands for consistency as a form of control and imprisonment. Out of anger, they may react to these patients as if their wishes for reliability and concern were infantile and irrational:

> Your complaints about my lateness are a reflection of your need to control me.

The psychiatrist's tardiness might in fact be creating tremendous anxiety because it reminds the patients of parents who never took their feelings into account.

Avoiding Dual Relationships

Psychiatrists should avoid treatment situations that place them in a conflict between therapeutic responsibility to patients and third parties. Examples of dual relationships in psychiatric practice include clinicians treating their own relatives and friends, the same therapist employing concurrent family and individual therapy paradigms with a given patient, and clinicians testifying as forensic witnesses for current psychotherapy patients.

Role conflicts are quite widespread and interfere with the practitioner's single-mindedness of purpose as a healer. Dual relationships interfere with the ability of psychiatrists to carry out their vital functions in the community.

The burgeoning expansion of prepaid care in the USA in the last two decades has provoked concern about a new source of role conflict for psychiatrists.

On the other hand, increasing coverage of the population of the USA under a system of managed care has generated serious concerns regarding potential conflicts of interest. This disquietude is particularly noticeable in the field of psychiatry. Although there is little scientific data to support the contention that restricted managed care panels are necessary for lowering costs, it is important that both patients and clinicians be informed about the hazard such a system of care entails. Since participation on a panel is often contingent on cost-efficiency profiles, psychiatrists who derive a significant portion of their income from a given managed care organization (MCO) are discouraged from advocating for patients needing more expensive care. In addition, some MCOs refuse to pay for integrated treatment for mentally ill patients by psychiatrists enrolled in their panel. Instead, these MCOs insist on a split treatment model in which the patient obtains psychotherapy from a social worker or psychologist and is allowed only brief medication management visits with a psychiatrist. Psychiatrists attempting to do medication management under this model often have little contact with the psychotherapist, are very restricted in the frequency and duration of visits with the patient, and are thereby limited in making overall clinical decisions that might become necessary. Such a situation creates an ethical bind for the psychiatrist in which the medical responsibility is not accompanied by a commensurate degree of authority to direct the treatment process.

Autonomy and Neutrality

Since the early days of modern psychotherapy, it has been recommended to adhere to a position of neutrality with patients by refraining from the temptation to take sides in the patient's internal conflicts or life problems. This advice has relevance for all psychiatric treatment, insofar as it espouses the idea that practitioners should maintain profound respect for their patients' autonomy and individuality. This is a fundamental therapeutic stance that fosters independence, growth, and self-esteem. It reinforces the idea that the clinician believes the patient to be the owner of his or her body, life, and problems. The patient receives the following message:

> The doctor tries to help by assisting me to learn about myself, not by trying to take control of me.

Cultural, ethnic, and probably sociodemographic factors strongly shape attitudes regarding patient autonomy and informed consent. In some cultures, a higher value may be placed on the harmonious functioning in the interlocking pattern of family relationships than on the autonomy of individual family members. The psychiatrist should diligently explore the role that cultural and family relationships play in the patient's healthy mental functioning and be guided primarily by the patient's communications about their degree of comfort or conflict with these family relationships. Psychiatrists should be considerate and respectful of cultural differences between themselves and their patients and be particularly cautious about interpreting those differences as a pathological process.

Mindful of cultural issues, indicated ways of encouraging autonomy include encouraging informed consent by outlining the potential benefits, risks, and alternatives for a proposed treatment approach; explaining the rationale for the treatment; and fostering the patient's participation in the treatment process. Acutely suicidal patients, however, often require the psychiatrist to assume temporary responsibility for their safety. Clinical actions that may interfere with the patient's autonomy include advice regarding nonurgent, major life decisions, attempting to exert undue influence on issues unrelated to the patient's health, reluctance to allow patients to terminate treatment, seeking gratification by exerting power over patients, and using power over patients as a form of retaliation.

Coherent and Noncollusive Compensation

Although there are rewards to be obtained from working in an interesting and creative profession, this is best applied to one's collective professional endeavors. When compensation is direct, there should be a set fee, and the patient should be responsible for the scheduled appointment time. When compensation is indirect or salaried, the psychiatrist must avoid colluding either with the patient against the party paying for the treatment or with the third party against the patient (see the previous section on avoiding dual relationships). Whatever method is being used for paying for mental health treatment, a coherent and noncollusive arrangement imparts the following message to the patient:

> The doctor has needs of his or her own, but they are limited to a salary or fee. Aside from financial obligations, I don't have to please, gratify, or nurture my doctor.

Generally risky compensation arrangements include working for a treatment organization one perceives to be financially exploitive, accepting inexpensive gifts from patients, especially when such gifts are not part of a culturally expected mode of behavior, bartering goods or services in return for treatment, referring patients for treatments or procedures in which one has a proprietary financial interest, and neglecting the patient's failure to adhere to the original agreement regarding payment of fees. Certain practices are absolutely contraindicated and likely to be destructive, including fraudulent billing, accepting expensive gifts, fee splitting, colluding with the patient or third party, and use of financial insider information.

Confidentiality

It is essential that psychiatrists treat their patients' communications as privileged. This means that patients alone retain the right to reveal information about themselves. The advent of managed care has raised even greater concern about the privacy of patients' personal communications with their psychiatrists because of the potential for an increasing number of persons connected with the MCO to have access to material from patients' files. Psychiatrists should caution their patient about the potential limitations to confidentiality and be prepared to explore the consequences of these exceptions. For example, if a patient is raising his or her mental health as an issue in litigation, some or all communications to a psychiatrist could be legally discoverable. Coherent boundaries with regard to confidentiality send the following message to the patient:

> My thoughts and feelings belong to me. The doctor does not treat them as if they belong to him or her.

Indicated means of preserving confidentiality include obtaining proper authorization from patients before releasing information, explaining the need for confidentiality with parents of children and adolescents, and involving all participants in family and group psychotherapy in agreements about confidentiality. Problematic activities that may endanger confidentiality include stray communications with concerned relatives of patients in individual psychotherapy, where there is no prior expectation on the patient's part about discussions with relatives; discussion of privileged information with the psychiatrist's own family members; releasing information about deceased patients; and failure to properly disguise case presentations.

Anonymity

Anonymity can be seen as a fundamental boundary issue applicable to all forms of psychiatric treatment. It serves as a reminder to both patient and clinician of the professional purpose of the relationship. Avoiding unnecessary personal disclosure to patients protects both patient and practitioner from a reversal of roles – one of the critical themes recurring in boundary violations. By maintaining a policy of relative anonymity, the patient receives the following message about the treatment:

> This is a place where I can bring my issues. The doctor doesn't burden me with his or her stuff.

Certain forms of self-disclosure are indicated in the course of work with psychiatric patients, including appraising patients of the clinician's qualifications and treatment methods as part of informed consent, discussing reality factors about the psychiatrist's health status or intentions regarding retirement that will impact on the patient's treatment decisions, and using "reality checks" to help patients contain disturbed and frightening fantasies.

Abstinence

Abstinence means that psychiatrists should discourage direct forms of pleasure such as touching or sexuality in the course of their interactions with patients. In the therapeutic relationship, the patient's ability to consent to sexual activity with the psychiatrist is vitiated by the knowledge the latter possesses over the patient and by the power differential that vests the psychiatrist with special authority.

For patients, actual gratification from the psychiatrist is best confined to realistic goals for recovery and emotional growth. Psychiatrists should limit themselves to the pleasure of getting paid for a job well done and for the opportunity to participate in an interesting and creative profession. Although steadfast application of this boundary can be quite frustrating for both doctor and patient, it pays excellent dividends in the long run by encouraging autonomy and a more mature way of dealing with impulses. The rule of abstinence as a therapeutic boundary has an analogous function to the incest taboo as a social organizer. From a practical standpoint, psychiatrists can strengthen their patients' boundaries in this regard by resisting behaviors such as physical touching, accepting gifts, socialization outside treatment, and sexual involvement. The patient receives the following messages from a clinician who is able to properly adhere to this principle:

> The doctor is more interested in my health than his or her own gratification and doesn't try to take possession of me. I am learning that I can have wishes that needn't result in action.

There are occasions when psychiatrists are obligated to employ physical procedures such as taking blood pressures, checking for extrapyramidal symptoms, restraining dangerous patients, or administering electroconvulsive therapy. Indeed, clinical touching of patients is considered an integral part of the physician–patient relationship because of its important role in physical examination and therapeutic procedures. Even though psychiatrists are physicians, they are obligated to use much more restraint in this regard than is expected of colleagues in other branches of medicine. It is probably too invasive for the same physician, on a protracted basis, simultaneously to intrude both into the patient's psychological and physical spaces.

Other risky forms of gratification include embracing or kissing patients, eating and drinking with patients, socializing with patients outside of the therapy setting, and failure to understand and resolve recurrent or obsessive sexual fantasies about a patient. Engaging in sexual behavior with current or former patients is contraindicated because it is almost invariably destructive, even though the damage may not be immediately manifest.

The APA (American Psychiatric Association, 1993) took a principled and unequivocal stand regarding sexual activity between psychiatrists and their current or former patients:

> Additionally, the inherent inequality in the doctor–patient relationship may lead to exploitation of the patient. Sexual activity with a current or former patient is unethical.

The APA's position is in agreement with the principles espoused in the Hippocratic Oath, which clearly mandates that a physician approach a patient "for the benefit of the sick, and … abstain from every voluntary act of mischief and corruption; and, further, from the seduction of females or males, of freemen and slaves".

Whether they realize it or not, psychiatrists who justify the permissibility of post-termination sexual relationships are sabotaging their own overlearned commitment to act primarily in their patient's best interest and are exposing their patient to a biased and error-prone treatment. This self-permissive attitude would make a psychiatrist more prone to engage in seductive grooming of a patient during the treatment process in anticipation of termination. In addition, biased by this attitude, a psychiatrist is likely to avoid making any communication to the patient that would discourage a subsequent romantic post-termination liaison (Epstein, 2002). While a psychiatrist might consciously deny that this attitude is a violation of the Hippocratic dictum, in actual cases where psychiatrists have engaged in post-termination sex with patients, their pretermination subliminal thinking ran like this:

> I'm treating this patient only for her or his benefit. Like Hippocrates, I will abstain from every voluntary act of mischief and corruption and, further, from seduction. However, after I cure this very attractive patient, I will keep his or her phone number, and after a respectable period of time, it will be a different matter, and we will see what will happen.

Note that this reasoning represents a form of dissociative thinking based on a primitive wish for inappropriate gratification with a patient that magically disavows the connection between posttreatment behavior and pretreatment reality. All psychiatric treatment is based on the assumption that a psychiatrist's interventions by means of positive attitudes, words, deeds, and medical interventions will have a lasting beneficial effect on the patient after the treatment has ended. There is no realistic escape from the fact that the reverse is also true, namely, that inappropriate attitudes, words, deeds, and interventions are likely to have a lasting harmful effect on the patient after the treatment has ended.

Self-respect and Self-protection

It is essential that psychiatrists protect themselves from being exploited by patients. This principle is necessary to protect clinicians and patients alike. Many patients seeking treatment have endured abusive relationships in which being victimized became the price for maintaining human connectedness. For such patients, efforts to exploit the psychiatrist may be an action–question that inquires:

> Must one of us be injured in order for us to have a close relationship?

By setting a proper role model for self-respect and self-caretaking, the psychiatrist imparts the following message to the patient:

> Relationships need not be structured on the basis that one or both parties must be exploited. If I as the doctor allow you to hurt me, I am setting a poor role model.

Psychiatrists should attempt to discuss the meaning of any exploitive behavior on the patient's part as soon as possible. With unstable or impulsive patients who are prone to acting out, confrontation should be timed to maximize safety. For example, it would be more prudent to interpret the manipulative aspects of a patient's suicidal behavior after the patient is admitted to a hospital. If a patient makes a sudden physical overture such as attempting a sexually provocative embrace, it must be dealt with the same urgency as a physical assault. The psychiatrist should inform the patient that such behavior is inconsistent with coherent treatment. It is generally risky to allow repeated exceptions such as last-minute prolongation of sessions, repeated lateness in paying fees, excessive intrusion into the psychiatrist's personal space in the form of regular and frequent late night phone calls, or taking items from the office.

Certain psychiatrists find themselves avoiding confrontation with an exploitive patient out of fear of the latter's narcissistic rage. This is an indication of an escalating situation that may lead to further boundary violations either by the patient or the psychiatrist.

Summary

The ethical and boundary issues discussed in this chapter were designed to stimulate a better understanding of an extremely thorny topic rather than to provide an exhaustive compendium. Table 8.5 summarizes selected indicators of potential boundary violations, along with remedial responses clinicians might employ to deal with these situations that

Table 8.5 Indicators of Potential Boundary Violations with Suggested Remedial Responses

Indicator	Suggested Remedial Response for Clinician
Clinician is frequently tardy starting sessions.	Avoid criticizing patient for complaining about lateness. Reexamine reasons for tardiness in light of patients' need for a stable treatment frame.
Clinician changes the treatment paradigm in "midstream", i.e., switching from individual therapy with Mr A to couples therapy with Mr A and his wife.	Avoid dual relationships that may interfere with primary loyalty to the first patient. If dual relationships cannot be avoided, explain risks to patient(s) according to principle of informed consent.

(Continued)

Table 8.5 *(Cont'd)*

Indicator	Suggested Remedial Response for Clinician
Clinician often relates to patient as if he or she were a personal friend.	Listen for signs that the patient feels burdened. Acknowledge pattern of role reversal and importance of clinician's fiduciary obligations to patient.
Clinician accepts gifts from patient.	Try to explore patient's motive for the gift. Consider refusing the gift by explaining that it might interfere with the effectiveness of treatment. Be prepared to work with patient's shame in this regard.
Clinician feels overly resentful about having to keep boundaries because they feel too constraining and spoil the "fun" and creativity of being a therapist.	Remember that therapy is hard work that is often burdensome and frustrating, and that boundaries are necessary for the patient's safety.
Clinician seeks contact with patient outside therapy setting.	Avoid contact, and explain the reason to patients. In settings where social contact is likely, discuss problems and options with the patient in advance.
Clinician is unable to confront patients who are late paying fees, remove items from the office, repeatedly try to prolong sessions, or torment therapist with insatiable demands.	Listen to the content of patient's communications and dreams regarding people injuring one another. Explore fear of one's own anger, the patient's anger, or of setting limits.
Clinician often tries to impress patients with personal information about himself or herself.	Refrain from further disclosure and examine one's possible motives. Consider how such activity might relate to sexual feelings to patient or need to control patient.
Clinician becomes sexually preoccupied with patient, for example, feels a pleasurable sense of excitement or longing when thinking of patient or anticipating his or her visit.	Consider that one's sexual feelings may portend the reenactment of an actual or symbolic incestuous scenario from the patient's past. Remember that incestuous behavior or its symbolic equivalent infantilizes the victim. Obtain supervision and/or personal psychotherapy if sexual preoccupations continue unabated.

some psychiatrists may encounter in keeping boundaries derived from many sources. It behoves psychiatrists to determine whether they have suffered deficiencies in training or adverse role modeling during the course of their professional development and whether their own emotional problems significantly interfere with maintaining coherent professional boundaries.

References

American Psychiatric Association (1973) Principles of medical ethics with annotations especially applicable to psychiatry. *American Journal of Psychiatry* 130, 1057–1064.

American Psychiatric Association (1993) *Principles of Medical Ethics with Annotations Especially Applicable to Psychiatry*. American Psychiatric Association, Washington, DC.

Epstein RS (1994) *Keeping Boundaries. Maintaining Safety and Integrity in the Psychotherapeutic Process*. American Psychiatric Press, Washington, DC.

Epstein RS (2002) Post-termination boundary issues (Letter). *American Journal of Psychiatry* 159, 877–878.

Goffman E (1974) *Frame Analysis. An Essay on the Organization of Experience*. Harvard University Press, Cambridge, MA.

Hippocrates (1929) *The Genuine Works of Hippocrates* (Trans. Adams F). William Wood, New York.

World Psychiatric Association Ethical Statements (2000) Appendix, in *Ethics, Culture and Psychiatry: International Perspectives* (eds Okasha A, Arboleda-Florez J and Sartorius N). American Psychiatric Press, Washington, DC, pp. 211–214.

Index